SO
YOU WANT TO OPEN A PROFITABLE DAY CARE CENTER

EVERYTHING YOU NEED TO KNOW TO PLAN, ORGANIZE AND IMPLEMENT A SUCCESSFUL PROGRAM

Patricia C. Gallagher

Young Sparrow Press
Box 265
Worcester, PA 19490
(215) 364-1945

With love
To my wonderful husband John
To my beautiful children:
Robin, Katelyn, Kristen and Ryan
To my loving parents Bob and Claire Mohan
and my family for their enthusiastic support

Published by YOUNG SPARROW PRESS

Box 265, Worcester, PA 19490 • 215-364-1945

Library of Congress Cataloging-in-Publication Data
Gallagher, Patricia C.
So You Want To Open A Profitable Day Care Center
Everything You Need To Know To Plan, Organize,
And Implement A Successful Program.
1. Day Care Centers 362.7   2. Day Nurseries
3. Child Care Business   4. Small Business
ISBN #0-943135-53-2 (pbk.)

Cover Design by Carrie J. Gamble

Cover Photography by Environments, Inc.,
Beaufort, South Carolina

Book Design by Kathleen M. Keiper, DeskTop Associates

Contents

PART THREE:
ASSESSMENT OF DAY CARE NEEDS

PART FOUR:
BUSINESS CONSIDERATIONS

PART FIVE:
ADMINISTRATION

PART SIX:
ADVERTISING AND PROMOTION

PART SEVEN:
ADVICE FROM THE EXPERTS

PART EIGHT:
EDUCATION CURRICULUM GUIDANCE

PART NINE:
CHILD SAFETY

PART TEN:
KEEPING STAFF & KIDS HAPPY

PART ELEVEN:
THE LEARNING ENVIRONMENT

APPENDICES

Preface

When I opened my first day care center in the early 1970's, its success had to have been fueled by my entrepreneurial enthusiasm alone! Although I had an undergraduate degree in Education and several years of experience as an elementary school teacher, I did not have the faintest idea of how to run a business.

I remember that it all happened rather quickly. Fortunately, things fell into place very easily and I opened the attractive, cheerfully-decorated child care center within three months. Insurance concerns and day care regulations were not difficult issues because mothers were not as prominent in the work force and day care was not the hot topic it is today. Realistically, taking such a project from start to completion in today's day care environment would take about a year.

As for me, I knew that 1) I loved children and teaching; 2) I had a high-energy level; 3) I wanted to start my own business; and 4) I was ready for a change from teaching in the school district.

How did I go about it?

Did I make a fortune?

Was it a rewarding experience or a disappointment?

What advice would I give to others now that I am fifteen years older and wiser?

Hopefully, in the pages that follow, you will learn by my mistakes and the "if I were to do it again" advice of the many day care center directors that were interviewed in researching this book. Yes, I earned a profit and found being a business owner to be a lot of fun, but I also learned the importance of many other factors that contribute to the success or failure of a business.

In addition to the experience of running a day care center, I also gained other pertinent experience and education. Graduate work in early childhood education enhanced my knowledge of child development, and a M.B.A. in finance aided in my understanding of management, accounting and the importance of the "bottom line."

This guidebook attempts to provide practical, easy-to-read, no-nonsense information that will assist entrepreneurs who are considering the operation of a day care business. It is quite an involved process but certainly not impossible to complete if you are aware of the possible stumbling blocks. I will share my experience and research on a variety of topics: licensing, obtaining occupancy permits, legal issues, special services, record keeping, health and safety, insurance, landlord and tenant relationships, advertising and promotion, etc. Factors contributing to the success of other programs will also be shared throughout this publication.

Related materials and resources are included so that simply by reading this book, you will be able to access additional free information. As a matter of fact, I advise you to sit down today and write out postcards to some of the selected resources on my list. Within a few weeks, your mailbox will be filled with excellent books, publications, catalogs and pamphlets.

In the appendices I have listed valuable sources of further information including federal agencies, small business administration offices, associations and organizations, magazines, newsletters and trade publications.

Don't hesitate to ask for help! I found that by calling various agencies listed in this book I was able to access information that is vital in the start-up and ongoing operation of a day care center.

I would like to thank the people who shared their wisdom and thus gave all of us the benefit of their experience. Some of the information which I have referred to in this publication was gleaned from manuals provided by various United States Government Printing Offices, Scotsman Buildings and Environments, Inc. A very special note of thanks to my editors, Cathy Skwara and Paula Dupont-Kidd, both cheerful perfectionists whose great care and commitment made this book possible.

Note: All information presented in this book is presented in good faith, thus no liability is assumed with respect to the use of information within. This book is not a substitute for child care and legal advice. The author and publisher assume no responsibility for errors, inaccuracies, omissions or any other inconsistencies within. In all matters related to opening a child care center, professionals such as consultants, accountants and attorneys should be consulted. You should refer to all statutes and regulations in your state, including legal and medical laws. In all matters relating to a child's health, particularly in respect to symptoms which may require diagnosis or medical attention, the parents and the child's physician should be consulted first.

Introduction

An Insider's View for Success

When I opened my first center, I was not married and had no children of my own. As a child care provider, I could offer care in a limited way. I had no way of really understanding the working mother's feelings of guilt, heartbreak upon hearing her child cry, feelings of sadness as she pulled away from the driveway, or annoyance when her child's clothing got mixed up or lost. Now, as a mother who has been on the other side of day care, I view things quite differently.

When I returned to work for AT&T as a marketing representative, I left my four-month-old daughter, Robin, in a day care arrangement. That experience really taught me the realities and dilemmas of the working parent. Now, I truly understand day care from both perspectives—the working parent and the child care provider.

Parents are interested in finding the perfect center. There is nothing more precious than your child. It is imperative to find caring people who will really love your child. I know that in a commercial business, where a profit and bottom line are important, it is easy to lose sight of the importance of nurturing and showing affection to the children. However, this is what parents want and what the children desperately need. The fast food restaurant-assembly line approach to child care will never do!

In your initial discussion with parents, try your best to understand the day care parent's dilemma. Try to feel their worry with them and assure them that their child will be special to you too! Answer their questions about homesickness, crying and clinging and explain the importance of a daily routine. Little children who are rushed by their parents to "Hurry up and eat," "Quick put your coat on," "C'mon, get in your car seat" are the product of an unpleasant morning routine. This will affect a child's adjustment to the day care experience. Of course, the evening pickup should be at a slower pace, even though it's tempting to rush a child to "Hurry, we have to go home."

Since most people who are considering opening a day care center have a background in teaching, nursing or social service, I have not focused heavily on curriculum planning. You probably have shelves of textbooks that can help you in that area. (Also, teacher's aid products and learning materials are introduced each year; you will want to keep abreast of the state-of-the-art innovations.) I have concentrated on the "how to's" of getting off to a good start, examining your motives, evaluating your experience and skills, advertising your business, establishing the ground rules, health and safety and troubleshooting information.

Your own experiences and special talents, combined with the practical suggestions offered in this book are what it takes to start and operate a profitable and successful day care business. I would suggest that you network with other day care directors, subscribe to trade magazines, attend conferences and read books and related articles.

Best of luck in this extremely rewarding and challenging venture!

On your mark, get set, go!

You are now the boss!

AUTHOR'S NOTE: Because the children in your care will be both boys and girls, I have chosen to use the pronoun "he" and "she" when referring to the children. I have used the neutral term "caregiver" when referring to adults throughout most of this book.

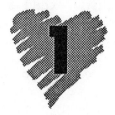

Agencies To Contact

WHERE DO I BEGIN?

There are three methods of starting a day care business. You can buy into a franchise, purchase an existing business or start your own "from scratch." There are definite pluses and minuses for each option. In this first section, we will discuss what is involved in starting your own, on your own, from square one. At the end of the chapter, you will find information about the other options.

Opening a day care center in an outside facility requires extensive planning and attention to detail. Once opened, it requires not only a good educational background but also strong business and management acumen. Most businesses fail because of poor record keeping and management practices. There are many books available in the library and bookstore that deal with starting a business. Even though they do not pertain to the day care business specifically, the principles are the same for most small business ventures. All businesses need start-up capital, have technicalities and legalities to understand and have to meet state regulations.

Contact the state's child care regulatory office which may be called the State Licensing Bureau, Department of Public Welfare, Social Services or Health and Human Services. (The appendix provides a complete listing.) Regulations vary from state to state and from community to community. Obtain a copy of the regulations and work hand-in-hand with your licensing representative.

Ask the representative if there are any training programs or orientations offered or if there are any subsidies or special incentives available for innovative programs. (If you care for low-income or subsidized day care families, special needs children, children with physical or mental disabilities, or incorporate adult day care with young children care, there may be special funding.)

The representative provides information about federal Title XX funds for subsidized care, welfare dollars for child care and the Child Care Food Program. The Child Care and Development Block grant provides federal funds to improve the quality of child care. The local government can use this money for a variety of purposes in the community. Check to see if any of this money supports child care and if money can be administered to help you start a center.

Request a list of the existing licensed day care homes and centers. Can the area support another center? Analyze the competition in terms of quality, fees charged, operating hours, etc.

Ask for the telephone number of the local Resource and Referral office. The local R&R may be able to assist you with becoming licensed when the process seems to be overwhelming. Their function is to recruit and train child care providers so there is ample available care for the community. They can tell you what types of care are frequently requested, where a new center should be located, and what age groups seem to be most in need of care. The National Association of Child Care Resource and Referral Agencies can provide information about the R&R agency in your area (see Appendix for address – phone #202-393-5501).

As you plan your center, network with others who have already been through the process and ask questions about: location, capacity, fees, insurance, health and safety practices, food, supplies and equipment, budget and record-keeping, relations with parents and activities. You will find the names of child care programs listed in the Yellow Pages. Look under: "child care," "day care," "day nurseries" and "nursery schools."

Contact the owner or director, although not one in your immediate area, and offer to pay a reasonable amount for a few hours of consulting. Your state licensing office can also provide a list of all the licensed programs in your state or county, thus by using such a list, you can contact directors for consulting. Experienced directors, owners and teachers often like to share their "war stories" as long as you are not in competition. Ask them to share their personal feelings on:

- Where can you obtain training in child development and early childhood education for staff?
- What is the optimal group size for infants, toddlers, preschoolers and school-age children?
- Is there a high turnover of caregivers and is this a big problem?
- Do you offer benefits to staff members?
- Any suggestions for retaining and hiring quality staff?
- How is equipment and space best arranged?
- Do they purchase food and supplies in bulk? Where?
- Any tips for establishing a good relationship with the parents?
- What advice would you give about waiting lists, hours, holidays, vacation schedules, fees, references and licensing?
- If you were to start over again, what would you do differently?

Ask for recommendations based on their experience.

Do not buy or lease a facility until you are certain that you can obtain a certificate of compliance from every regulatory entity. For example, in addition to state regulations, you need local zoning approval or a special municipal provision must be observed. This type of local approval may be over and beyond what is mandated by the state licensing bureau. Unless you have a signed operating certificate from each agency, you will not be permitted to operate or could be closed down after opening for failure to comply.

The licensing bureau provides a booklet that explains general requirements about the following: standards for staffing ratios, responsibilities, qualifications, building and physical site considerations, equipment, recommended programs for children, forms for staff and child health appraisal, food and nutrition, transportation, procedures for application and admission of children, child and employee record keeping, special program requirements and special exceptions to regulations, which are called waivers. (Read and reread!) Beware of easy to miss regulations! Some states prohibit two-story structures or require an exit door from every classroom. Some requirements may include allocating parking spaces or erecting fences. Each state has its own requirements—find out who you can contact for advice in your own licensing bureau.

The state child care monitor will probably provide you with a "to-do" checklist of the county or city agencies that you must notify of your intent. In other words, file the forms, pay the fees and heed the regulations. Find out which permits have to be renewed annually and ask about how long the process takes for approving a permit.

A sampling of the optimal ratios of adult to children is listed below. Children thrive when more adults are present than required by the state mandate. All adults should be kind, patient and responsible. This ratio is used by some states. It does not apply nationwide as each state sets its own standards. You must contact the licensing office in your state about the standards that you must meet to operate a licensed center. In some states, the ratios are as follows:

> one adult for every three to four infants and toddlers
> one adult for every four to six two-year-olds
> one adult for every seven to eight three-year-olds
> one adult for every eight to nine four-year-olds
> one adult for every eight to ten five-year-olds
> one adult for every ten to twelve after-school children

The National Association for the Education of Young Children (NAEYC) offers an accreditation program for day care centers. The key elements necessary to attaining this accreditation are: staff structure, staff training, interactions between children and providers, cleanliness, safety and adequate age-appropriate equipment. Call 800-424-2460 to request information.

In addition to the state regulations, there are other additional operating permits to be obtained.

1. **The zoning bureau or property zoning bureau** in your city has ordinances that determine what types of businesses may operate in a particular area. You may find out who governs this by calling the city hall, police, mayor's office, city council or superintendent's office. Be sure to inquire what taxes must be paid on a particular location. You may be surprised that some taxes are more exorbitant than you expected and in turn make a particular location unattractive.

Before making any final decisions about purchasing or leasing a building, be certain the zoning official has stated in writing that the building is approved as a day care center location. If it is not, a public hearing may be needed to obtain a special permit or variance. If a variance is required, a non-refundable application fee for filing is charged. My advice is that fighting for the location is usually a waste of time and money. Don't fight for a location that the people in the township are against. It will create bad feelings before you even begin and you may not be able to attract customers.

If you wish to renovate, add an addition or make any changes to the existing site, be sure that the zoning board has approved your plans in writing. IMPORTANT: A competent attorney should be involved with the zoning issue and should write a clause into any lease or purchase contract that will allow you to dissolve any agreement should your plans fall through and you are not able to proceed with opening the day care center. Just because it is zoned for day care does not mean that it will meet all of the requirements for final day care approval! The zoning approval is just one piece of the demanding puzzle. You may want to inquire if there are special restrictions in the township about day care centers. Over and over again, I have heard of problems regarding restrictions on type, placement, size and number of signs permitted in front of a center.

You may call NAEYC (National Association for the Education of Young Children), 800-424-2460, and ask for their catalog of day care related publications, one of which deals very heavily with the zoning issue. Some of the issues you'll need to understand are: what is zoning, state zoning enabling laws, zoning classifications, the typical ordinance, zoning treatment of day care, zoning flexibility, obtaining zoning flexibility for day care, improving the zoning status of day care, etc. Ask which publication they would recommend to help you with the legal aspects of day care center organization and operation.

2. **Building Code Inspections,** usually administered by the Department of Building Safety or the County Building Department, are required before a permit of approval is issued. It is imperative that the facility is deemed safe for children. The inspector will be concerned with the conditions of building construction, ventilator fans, radiators, heating, electrical and plumbing systems, level of asbestos and lead paint, emergency exits, screens on windows, emergency lighting, etc. Before agreeing to a building site, ask yourself some honest questions. Even if you believe it is feasible to modify, renovate or fix some of the above areas, is it advantageous to you cost-wise? Ask about the number of blueprints required to file, application fees, etc. Be sure to have a preliminary inspection by all agencies before you buy, lease or agree to use any facility.

3. **Fire Safety Approval** must be obtained. The local department will survey the building and guide you as to the requirements: alarms, fire extinguishers (which must be recharged periodically), fire drill plans, the number and type of fire doors, type of roof, walls and floor coverings. Be prepared for periodic inspections by the fire marshal. You will have to keep a fire drill log that is dated to indicate that you practice emergency

procedures with the children. Ask the fire fighting professionals for advice on emergency procedures in the event of fire, tornadoes, storms, gas leaks, blackouts and chemical spills which could occur without warning. (Do you have easy access for emergency vehicles?)

4. **Licensing and Inspections,** often referred to as L&I, is a regulatory agency that inspects for conditions of electrical and plumbing systems, general building construction, number of exits, health and safety procedures. Ask your state licensing representative to provide you with a list of all agencies that you should contact for the wide range of approvals. Ask in what order you should go about obtaining permits. Ask if permits are contingent upon obtaining other permits. Ask where should you go first, second, third, etc. There is some overlap of regulation among the bureaus.

5. **The Sanitation and Board of Health Bureaus,** sometimes known as the State Health Department, approval may be required if you serve food. All food service personnel should possess a health card or statement of health from the local health department or physician. Some states do not send inspectors to check facilities for compliance with local state standards. In such a situation, you should designate a person with knowledge of applicable sanitation laws and regulations who should check annually for compliance with these regulations and be responsible for the correction of existing violations. You should be able to provide written evidence of this. Self-inspection reports should be completed to assure maintenance of standards. The following areas should be addressed: cleanliness and safety of food before, during and after preparation, including maintenance of correct temperature; cleanliness and maintenance of food preparation, service, storage, and delivery areas and equipment; insect and rodent control; garbage disposal methods; dish-washing procedures and kitchen equipment; food handling practices; health of food service personnel; water supply (be especially careful if you are using well water and do not have public sewer and water). Local or state sanitarians in health agencies can be most helpful in providing ideas on ways to meet sanitation standards. Contact Child Nutrition Division, Food and Nutrition Service, USDA, 3101 Park Center Drive, Alexandria, VA 22302 for materials and information on food programs. They provide suggested sources of menus and recipes for cooking and serving large quantities of food. Tested recipes are recommended to insure uniform quality, prevent waste and serve as a guide to purchasing. Other needed records include food and equipment inventories, personnel evaluation and training records.

6. **The Federal Food Program,** called the Child Care Food Program, is run by the Department of Agriculture and administered by sponsoring agencies. CCFP provides food money for some centers. There is an income-eligibility requirement for center-based programs. Ask if money is allocated to centers, the application procedure and the income level requirements for receiving free or reduced-fee meals and snacks. If you plan to serve food, you will receive helpful information from this organization. This

agency is interested in the cleanliness of bathroom and kitchen facilities. In some states, you may be required to hire a dietician or cook. The dietician should be knowledgeable about appropriate portions for children's servings and balanced meal plans for the parents to review. Due to cultural and religious variables, you may be asked to provide special dietary considerations for some children. The Board of Health will scrutinize your storage areas, food preparation methods, waste disposal and means of ventilation. If the cost of renovating a kitchen to serve meals is prohibitive or if you would prefer not to get involved with food preparation, each child could bring a lunch. For information about the food program, contact your licensing bureau, the local resource and referral agency, the State Department of Education or the Bureau of Nutrition.

BUYING AN EXISTING
DAY CARE CENTER BUSINESS

There are several sources to search to find established day care centers for sale. The following are some suggested sources:
- newspaper classified ads
- business, real estate brokers and bankers
- State Child Care Licensing Bureau
- Small Business Administration liquidation officer
- insurance agents
- day care owner networking meetings
- friends
- relatives
- day care centers in which you are interested
- Better Business Bureaus
- Chamber of Commerce

Don't be over anxious. Often when people wish to sell or unload, the reason for selling is listed as either the owner is retiring, has personal problems or a family member is in poor health. One of the reasons may be true but lurking in the background could be other problems of a more serious nature. Non-compliance with building and government codes, violations of health and licensing department ordinances, unethical business practices, a declining enrollment, or the owner's frustration with parents, staff and kids could potentially cause problems for you. It is important to protect yourself against problems such as a pending lawsuit, a leaking roof or a building needing major repair. Don't rush in to what appears to be a deal. The financial records that are shown to you or the seller's claims about profitability will probably make everything appear OK. No doubt, they will indicate that they are making a profit, have full enrollment and maintain a reliable staff. But beneath the surface, you must investigate the physical facility, the equipment, reputation, etc. With a suspicious eye and a sharp mind, take note. What equipment needs to be repaired or replaced? Check with the above listed agencies to be sure that they have been inspected recently and do not have any citations against them. Inquire at the Better Business Bureau and the Chamber of Commerce for possible reasons for the sale. Ask around the neighborhood to determine the public opinion of the existing center. Is it well thought of? What is included in the business agreement—customer lists, signs, shelving, desks, furniture, fixtures and equipment?

Make a reasonable offer. Don't overpay. Remember that the owner probably really wants to get rid of the business so you have the advantage in negotiating. There is probably not a large demand to purchase this type of investment. Agree in writing that the current owner will be available to spend a specified number of hours sharing ideas and opinions on what worked and what didn't regarding advertising through the mail, Yellow Pages, flyers and daily newspapers. Have honest discussions about pricing, policy and the competition. You do not want to reinvent the wheel. Establish rapport so that they share information. Put everything in writing. Review all contracts with an accountant and attorney so that full disclosure of all representations, conditions, obligations, debts, terms and conditions are assured.

Be sure to sign a "non-compete clause," also known as a "covenant not to compete," so that the owner does not open a beautiful, new expanded facility down the street, thus taking business away from you. On the positive side—an existing center is ready to go when you buy it from someone else. The customers are in place, the reputation is established and the equipment is set up.

BE PATIENT! DO ALL OF YOUR HOMEWORK BEFORE SIGNING ON THE DOTTED LINE OF A CONTRACT! PROCEED WITH CAUTION.

CONSIDERATIONS ABOUT FRANCHISES

Opportunities abound for franchising in businesses such as ice cream parlors, muffler shops, car rental companies and child care centers. The advantages of franchises are: an established name, logo or slogan; design and set up of interior; marketing experience of the franchisor; and immediate familiarity with business procedures. An on-site or corporate training session complete with a manual developed by the franchisor helps with the start-up phase and on-going operation. There is usually a one-time fee, payable in advance, plus the cost of equipment and supplies. Expect ongoing royalty payments made to the parent company. Watch out for schemes, scams and franchisors who may not be available to keep their promises in the future.

Before buying a franchise, read books on the subject and talk to anyone who has ever purchased a franchise. Quick print shop proprietors, laundromat owners or ice cream parlor franchisees may offer good insight. Ask how they feel about fees and other franchise costs, the amount of support promised and in reality delivered, hidden fees and the total performance of the franchise operation.

There are several day care franchising opportunities available. Talk, and if possible, visit with existing franchise owners. Try to get in touch with ones who have gone out of business. Franchise agreements are quite complicated and restrictive. You need the counsel of a lawyer and CPA before signing a franchise agreement. *The Franchise Opportunities Handbook* is available for a fee from the Superintendent of Documents, U.S. Government Printing Office, Washington, D.C. 20402. LOOK BEFORE YOU LEAP! BEWARE OF OVERZEALOUS AND AMBITIOUS FRANCHISE SALES REPRESENTATIVES.

CONSIDERATIONS ABOUT HIRING A CHILD CARE CONSULTANT

As with any business, a knowledgeable professional can make the process easier ... but costlier. Before hiring a consultant, check references and experience, match the consultant's services to your goals and agree on a timetable and fee for the project in writing. Scotsman Buildings offers the following advice in their publication, *A Comprehensive Approach to Child Care Facilities.*

Many organizations and individuals who are considering opening a child care center have little direct experience in the field. Others who are knowledgeable about child care are totally inexperienced in needs assessment, financing, real estate and public relations—to name just a few areas where outside advice might be helpful. Using the services of a child care consultant with expertise in areas you may be lacking can save months in preparation and recoup the cost several times over.

Other areas where a consultant can help are site evaluation; interior design and space planning; licensing; management; staffing and curriculum. The services you need from a consultant may range from simply providing advice during the early stages of your project to monitoring the entire project through completion, and even managing the center once it is in operation. To get in touch with consultants, contact: the Association of Child Care Consultants International, 109 S. Bloodworth Street, Raleigh, NC 27601(919) 834-6506 or NAEYC, 1834 Connecticut Avenue, N.W., Washington, DC 20009, 800-424-2460. Don't overlook hiring the services of another experienced day care owner in your area.

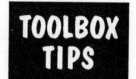

Starting a business is risky at best; but your chances of making it go will be better if you understand the problems you'll meet and work out as many of them as you can before you start.

U.S. Small Business Administration

Professionals To Contact

First, you must establish that you have the skills, energy, experience and education to open a day care center. Have you studied the rules and regulations required in your state? Then, it is time to select experienced professionals who can guide you through the maze of legalities. Issues such as signing a lease, securing licenses and adequate insurance, planning a bookkeeping system and discussing banking issues can be confusing for the new business owner. Once again, read all that you can about operating a business and then armed with this knowledge, select professionals to help you. Network with others and ask their opinion about recommendations for competent and reliable professionals. Agree on the fees you will pay for services ahead of time. You need to know whether you will be charged an hourly fee, an annual retainer fee for day-to-day services or a flat monthly charge. You need to know what additional costs are involved for litigation and other major services.

ACCOUNTANTS

A certified public accountant is absolutely necessary. Choose one that is recommended to you by another successful day care center director. Don't select one at random from a newspaper ad or the phone book. Make an appointment to discuss all registrations, forms and procedures that must be understood. You need professional help for many services including: determining your business structure, registration of the business with the city and county to receive an occupancy license, applying for a federal tax identification number, etc. (The federal tax identification number is needed in order to comply with tax regulations involving F.I.C.A. and federal income tax withholding procedures.) If you are not run by a government agency, an organizational structure must be determined (sole proprietorship, partnership, corporation). Your tax status will be determined by the type of organizational structure selected.

Ask your accountant to recommend a daily workbook system to help monitor cash-in and cash-out. Most office supply stores sell pre-printed record keeping journals. Keep good financial records so that you utilize your accountant's financial and tax law expertise more wisely, rather than paying him/her for organizing your records.

Your accountant will advise you to save receipts for everything. Tax laws change annually and therefore you should track in a systematic fashion all of your operating expenses such as: rent, supplies, salaries, advertising, insurance, taxes, utilities, depreciation, travel, accounting services and miscellaneous. All monies spent for transportation, mileage, equipment, food, gifts, supplies, professional journals, trade magazines, newsletters, educational conferences, parties should be categorized.

Ask your accountant how to handle the periodic tax returns that employers are required to file monthly, quarterly or annually to the government. The annual tax return is required whether you are profit or non-profit and whether you have made or lost money. Be sure to clarify what functions will be performed by the accountant and agree on a reasonable fee ahead of time.

Other examples of IRS requirements that you should be aware of include:

■ **Withholding Exemption Certificate**

You probably remember the forms that you filled out when you started a new job. This certificate determines how much tax is withheld for federal, state and city income taxes. Forms are obtained from the IRS office and are needed for each of your employees.

■ **Not-for-Profit Centers**

Such organizations are required to file detailed financial reports. If you are operating under this status, understand the procedures so that you do not incur a penalty or loss of license. Profit-making centers and non-profit centers are treated differently by the IRS. In a profit-making center, the parents' fees provide the income. A not-for-profit center receives money from the government or a philanthropic source.

■ **Federal Unemployment Compensation**

You contribute money into this fund for your employees. If you fire someone or lay them off, they may have the right to collect from this fund.

LAWYERS

A lawyer with good, honest, previous proven experience with day care issues is vital to the success of your center. (The lawyer who handled a friend's divorce may not have expertise in the day care field!) In addition to helping you determine the organizational form or legal structure such as sole proprietorship, partnership, corporation, profit or not-for-profit, this expert can explain all of the intricacies about liability. There are issues such as financial liability and personal liability. We live in a litigious society. People who believe that they were wronged sue readily so you want to understand liability.

Your lawyer can also advise you about hiring practices and personnel. There are questions that you are not permitted by law to ask prospective employees. It may be a sticky issue to question employment candidates about height, weight, sexual preferences, age, religion, race, etc. So that you are not faced with a discrimination lawsuit, seek the advice of your lawyer as it pertains to hiring and personnel practices.

Note: Some of the information you'll need to start your center overlaps in areas and you don't want to pay two professionals to perform the same function. If possible, schedule a meeting with the lawyer and accountant at the same time.

Your lawyer or accountant can help you with business requirements such as obtaining:

■ **Employer Identification Number**

This is required when you hire salaried employees. Forms are available from the IRS. These are free and are not complicated.

■ **State Unemployment Insurance** (Department of Employment Security or Department of Unemployment Compensation)

Most states require forms that pose questions about your employees, tax status, type of business, etc. As an employer, you contribute to a fund that will be used as unemployment compensation if your employees are not working and are given unemployment benefits. This procedure is handled differently for profit and non-profit businesses.

■ **Social Security**

As an employer, you will have to pay Federal Insurance Contribution Act (FICA) tax. This is a tax which is deducted from an employee's paycheck in a percentage amount that must be matched by the employer. (Non-profit centers are handled differently.)

INSURANCE PROVIDERS

Finding an insurance broker experienced with day care can be extremely critical. So many accidents are possible. You need this protection for yourself, your staff, volunteers, visitors, etc. Since there are many types of insurance coverages, a licensing representative can tell you first what is required. A word of caution here—what is required may be a minimal amount, but not adequate enough to protect your business interests. Investigate the options to find the policy that best meets your needs and budget. Some companies offer packages for medical, health and life insurance. Make sure that you obtain adequate liability insurance to protect you against lawsuits!

Develop a clear understanding of the following types of insurance: liability, health and medical for children and staff, automobile, transportation, fire, theft, workmen's compensation, Fidelity Bonds (available to protect against financial wrongdoing by day care center employees), business interruption insurance, extended coverage for storm and explosion damage and life insurance.

You certainly do not need all types of insurance. A good agent, who has your best interests at heart, will write the policy so that you are not going broke paying high insurance premiums. Insurance is a complex subject and can be quite costly. I would advise you to talk to other center owners, child care providers, local licensing offices and professional organizations for their input. The following sources can help you with insurance information. This list does not imply an endorsement or a recommendation, but is provided as a starting point for obtaining insurance coverage.

National Association for the Education of Young Children (NAEYC)
1834 Connecticut Avenue, NW
Washington, D.C. 20009
800-424-2460

Insurance Information Institute
1110 Williams Street
New York, NY 10038
212-669-9200

Human Services Risk Management
818 E. 53rd Street
Austin, TX 78751
800-222-4051

Child Care Information Exchange
Box 2890
Redmond, WA 98073
206-883-9394

Forrest T. Jones & Co.
3130 Broadway
Box 418131
Kansas City, MO 64141-9131
1-800-821-7303

CIGNA Corporation
2 Liberty Place
1601 Chestnut St.
Philadelphia, PA 19192
800-238-2525

The key is to shop around, not necessarily for the best price, but for sufficient coverage at a reasonable premium. You need insurance for peace of mind and as protection from a potential major loss. Keep your center free of safety hazards, hire responsible help and maintain adequate insurance coverage at all times.

As a child care professional, you should become a member of NAEYC. It is not at all expensive. You will receive a variety of publications, special member privileges and will be advised of conferences—both nationally and locally. Contact NAEYC and ask for the chapter in your area. Call for information and attend a few meetings before actually joining. This is a great way to learn sources for selecting the professionals listed above.

WHAT TYPES OF INCIDENTS/ACCIDENTS CAN HAPPEN?

In confidential conversations with day care owners and teachers, the following incidents were relayed to me. Accidents and incidents can and do happen but as you can see from the list below, some of the accidents indicate a lack of adequate supervision and could have been avoided.

- A baby bottle warmer with scalding hot water fell on a child.
- Several fingers were pinched in a swing set.
- A hand was crushed in a door that was slammed shut.
- A child walked behind a transportation van and was hit.
- The teacher left one preschooler at the zoo.
- A toy shelf not bolted to the wall fell on a child causing severe head

injuries.
- A child drowned in a swimming pool.
- A toy box lid slammed shut and the child's neck was broken.
- A driver left a group of children in a van while she went into a bank.
- A child choked on a hot dog.
- A child fell while running with a pencil and punctured his cheek.
- A door leading to the street was left unlocked and a child left the facility without anyone's knowledge.
- Inadequate refrigeration of food led to spoilage which in turn sickened an entire center of fifty children.
- A mother and child fell on a slippery sidewalk outside of the center.
- A baby fell from a changing table.

SMALL BUSINESS CONSULTANTS

A small business consultant can be accessed by calling your local Small Business Administration office. The Small Business Administration's national headquarters is located at: SBA, Office of Consumer Affairs, 1441 L Street, N.W., Room 503-D, Washington, D.C. 20416, (800-827-5722). The SBA provides workshops, courses and literature. A sub-group of the SBA is SCORE, which is the Service Corp. Of Retired Executives. Their services are low cost or no cost. See the appendix for information for the office nearest to you. The Small Business Development Center, also sponsored by the SBA, provides assistance to small businesses. In each state, there are offices at colleges, universities and state offices. They provide technical and management assistance. They are definitely worth looking into. Also contact the local Chamber of Commerce for requirements for starting a business. The MBA programs at many universities offer the services of their students as consultants and researchers. They sometimes are assigned to help you as part of a project which they will be graded on. Also check the telephone directory for government office listings that pertain to day care services. Tell people what you are doing and ask for their advice.

CAUTIONS ABOUT LEASING CONTRACTS

Despite all the advice the "professionals" will provide, you still will make the final decisions. Caution is needed in all business transactions, but especially those with long-term effects. Leasing contracts are one of those areas. Therefore, before signing an agreement for a lease, inquire about the former tenants in this location. You need to ask these questions:

Why did they leave?
Did they go out of business?
Was the landlord difficult to get along with?
Will the landlord permit a day care center in this location?
Is the area zoned for day care?
Is the location in a low traffic area?
Is the parking adequate?

Is the building up to all codes and ordinances?

What are the utility costs?

Are you responsible for utility payments, or is that included in your rent?

If there has been a high turnover in a particular location and there are a lot of vacancies in a particular area, you should re-evaluate your site selection.

Read the fine print of the lease agreement to be sure that there are no restrictions for operating a day care business.

Utilities often charge commercial business rates and private home rates. Find out which you would be paying. You might be surprised at the difference in charges.

If you are new to this business, my advice would be to sign a one- or two-year lease with an option for renewal. Your business may be an overwhelming success or you may realize that there are some shortcomings that you did not anticipate. Your own personal situation could change too. You could marry, divorce or move to another state and a long-term lease of five or ten years would be a legal commitment obliging you to continue payments long after your center discontinued services.

Negotiate the points in a lease agreement. Ask for concessions if the existing lease is not favorable to you.

Here is a checklist of some other questions you should ask regarding signing a lease:

- When will the rent be increased?
- How and when is the rent to be paid?
- Are increases scheduled or is the rate firm for the term of the lease?
- Is there an option to renew?
- Who is responsible for lawn care, snow removal, plumbing, wiring, roof repairs, extermination, garbage removal, insurance and any increases in real estate tax?
- Exactly what areas of the building and outdoor space can be used?
- Can you use the building after hours for parent or staff meetings?
- Is the lease transferable?
- Must you carry insurance?
- If it is a church property, can you use the playground, church Bible School equipment, etc.?

My own learning experience was a percentage rent clause or "catch clause" written into the fine print of our lease agreement. The landlord not only received a monthly payment but also required a copy of our financial statements at year's end to collect a percentage of our gross income, which really entitled him to higher rent from us. Of course, upon this discovery, we terminated our lease at the end of our legal obligations. This is common in a space rented in a shopping center.

Be sure that an attorney reviews the lease and assists you in all negotiations related to complex lease agreements. There are many types of leases. A clause of "pending approval" should be included in the negotiated document.

None of the above information should be taken too lightly. Remember to work very closely with your state licensing representative so that all bases are covered. Do not sign anything unless your lawyer has written in a contingency stating that all contracts, deals and agreements are null and void if appropriate permits are not obtainable. Hire the services of competent professionals before you begin so that you don't have unexpected problems later on.

In many cases, you can obtain waivers to bypass certain regulations if you agree to complex and expensive changes. But remember a day care center is not the easiest way to make a million dollars so be careful about how you spend your money. Many departments and consulting experts will charge reviewing and filing fees. Another factor is that licenses expire periodically, so be sure to have a renewal filing system in place so you can reapply without incurring penalties and experiencing problems.

IMPORTANT:

Please use this manual as a guide book only. Check and recheck local and state regulations since they are subject to many changes. Use the services of professionals to assist you. Also use your own good judgement when it comes to safety. You, alone, know your particular situation and what is best for your center and the children in your care.

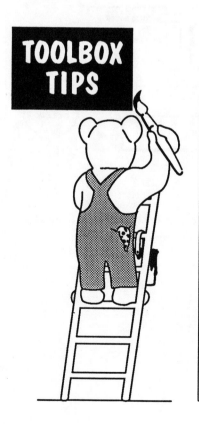

TOOLBOX TIPS

"You never get a second chance to make a first impression. Within the first 60 seconds on the telephone and five minutes on a center tour, child care prospects form an impression of you that is often a lasting one. The image you project determines to a great extent whether or not your prospects enroll, your customers stay, and the opinion influencers in the community refer you and your child care services."

Marketing Letter for Child Care Professionals
Credit: Julie Wassom, Editor, The Enrollment Generator

Typical Approval Process for a Child Care Center

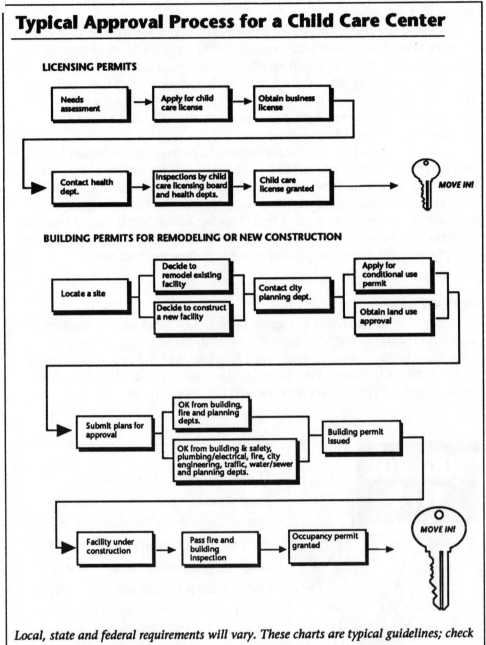

LICENSING PERMITS

Needs assessment → Apply for child care license → Obtain business license

Contact health dept. → Inspections by child care licensing board and health depts. → Child care license granted → **MOVE IN!**

BUILDING PERMITS FOR REMODELING OR NEW CONSTRUCTION

Locate a site → Decide to remodel existing facility / Decide to construct a new facility → Contact city planning dept. → Apply for conditional use permit / Obtain land use approval

Submit plans for approval → OK from building, fire and planning depts. / OK from building & safety, plumbing/electrical, fire, city engineering, traffic, water/sewer and planning depts. → Building permit issued

Facility under construction → Pass fire and building inspection → Occupancy permit granted → **MOVE IN!**

Local, state and federal requirements will vary. These charts are typical guidelines; check with the local governing authorities for the regulations of your community.
Credit: Scotsman Buildings

Assessment Of Day Care Needs

Many new business owners are excited when they see a potential site that appears to be all that they desired in a day care center location. Although, at first glance, the space for a playground is ideal and the building appears in tip-top shape, there are important issues to consider before plunging ahead.

Research, analyze and study these issues:

1. Is there a need for day care in the community?
   How many centers are already in operation?
   The parents may need day care in the community,
   but can they afford to pay for your type of program?

2. Where should I locate?
   Consider a high growth area where shopping malls, factories, plants, office buildings and industries are firmly established or on the increase. Possibly select an area where young professionals live and work. Contact the Chamber of Commerce, the local library or the business department of a university for business information. Perhaps a student recently did a term paper on the day care demographics and you can take advantage of the study.

3. Is there a large pre-school population?
   What age group seems to be most in need of care?
   Drive through the neighborhood and observe. Be sure that there are enough people in the area to support this kind of business. Call the Census Bureau. Find out the number of working families with children from infancy to age six. The licensing bureau knows the needs of the community. Ask at the elementary school about the number of children living in the area who need after-school care. Find out if there are waiting lists at other centers for a particular age group. That may be the group

most in need of care in your area.

4. What type of program is needed and what do you wish to offer?
   Is there a niche that has not been filled?

Although there may be several centers in the area, you may cater to the needs of a special group. Think about your philosophy. Will you stress religion, academics, play? Understand your target market. Ascertain that they are willing and able to afford any special services that you offer.

5. Will a lot of traffic go past the day care center?

Your center will be visible to large numbers of people if there is a large retail store or food store nearby. Also, well-known stores tend to draw people to the area. Ask business owners in the area what they think of your proposed location.

6. Is the driveway easy to enter and exit for the parents?
   Is there ample parking?

7. Is the location "on the beaten track?"

Parents want the center to be convenient. Sites that are located near major highways, bus depots, residential areas and public transportation are preferable. Locations near a university, military base, shopping mall, etc., can cater to the needs of the parents who are employed in such places and can provide a steady stream of new business.

8. Are windows, frontage and the layout of the building adequate to advertise your business?

Window displays, lighting and a playground are ways to draw attention to your center. In real estate promotion, the key phrase is "location, location, location." Parents are looking for convenience either close to home, close to work, or enroute to work. They want to be able to get in and out of traffic easily. With all of the pressures of maintaining a home and work schedule, parents are reluctant to go off the beaten track to drive to a day care center. Also, a brightly decorated, attractive facility, playground or sign is one of your best and least expensive forms of advertising. If you are located where the traffic pattern is light, you will be missing a good chance to show off your playground filled with happy children and enthusiastic staff.

HOW DO I FIND A POTENTIAL SITE?

Drive around the area you wish to consider for a day care operation. Look for day care centers that are in operation. Perhaps you could do this on a Sunday when the centers are closed. The telephone book or the state list of centers provides the names and addresses. Walk around the property. Peek in the windows. Analyze the "curb appeal." To a parent riding by, what is attractive and what detracts from a favorable impression? Jot down what you like and don't like. What do they have in the playground? How about the type of fence? Now you have an idea of what other centers offer in the area. Do you like the center located in a church, school, apartment complex, corporation? What are the pros and cons of each location?

Start by contacting the city housing authority, zoning board and real estate offices. Ask if they know of any buildings that may be suitable or may soon become available. Any homes, apartments, condominiums for rent or sale? Remember, they are not cognizant of all that is involved with day care regulations and local ordinances regarding day care specifically. Consider their suggested locations as possible leads only. One real estate representative showed a home to a prospective day care center owner. She pointed out that it was perfect for a center because it was on a main thoroughfare, had a great parking lot, an enclosed yard and lots of space for happy little children. Unfortunately, after the settlement papers were completed, the heartache began. Although it appeared to be a perfect location to the realtor and the inexperienced day care operator, the site was not acceptable. Over $150,000 had been paid for a large home that was not approved by the various regulatory agencies. The problem was an underground sewage system. The existing sewer facility did not have the capacity to handle the needs of fifty children and the staff. The cost to fight this issue and install a new sewer system was out of the question. A check with the local public works department would have provided information about this stumbling block, but most people would not even give a thought to sewers, water mains and hook-ups for utilities.

After selecting four possibilities, ask the licensing representative to give an opinion of each location. Some possible sites are: large house, vacated school building, factory, nursing home, hospital, church, synagogue, single story apartment complex or unit, community building, corporation, retail store, college campus, military facility or government office building. Ask about the pros and cons of each of the above locations. Be sure that the condition of the potential site is in sufficient state of repair in regard to sturdy construction of walls, floors and ceilings.

Contact ministers, rabbis and priests to see if they have space that they would like to donate or make available at a reduced rate. Ask school superintendents and principals if there are any empty classrooms. Once again, the location must meet stringent requirements whether it is located in an empty school building, private industry, church or retail shop.

Let the buyer beware is important in this business. Beware of ads in the paper that someone is selling their center! Investigate as to why. I know of someone who was selling because a local inspector told her that she needed extensive electrical work done to the property. She decided to "unload"—leaving the problem for an unsuspecting new owner. She told the buyer that her family was going to purchase a new business opportunity. You guessed it. She opened another nicer center three miles away!

Ask businesses in the area what they think of your proposed site selection. They may be aware of the main road being closed for construction in the near future, thus inconveniencing parents and cutting all opportunities for drive-by visibility for advertising purposes. An area business owner may be aware that your potential location is near a large sinkhole or that at certain times of the year, there is a very foul smell that reeks from a plant nearby.

On the positive side, suppose business really booms. Would you be permitted to expand at this location? For example, the zoning board may not permit further building on this site.

As you can see, you must be a thorough detective when investigating your center's potential location, clientele and opportunity for success!

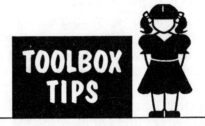

TOOLBOX TIPS

"As employer sponsored child care receives more attention in the media, it is seen as a new option for employment for child care professionals. Thus the deluge from new consultants who attempt, often without the necessary experience, to develop quality options for children. To work in child care settings does not give someone the necessary credentials to establish programs within a corporate setting. These consultants are well intentioned but naive."

Credit: Anne Cairns Federlein, Ph.D., Expert in Child Care Trends

Business Considerations

WHAT IS THE PROFIT POTENTIAL OF THIS BUSINESS?

There are many variables that affect profits. Since day care is an issue for the future, there should be a constant demand for these services. Some of the factors that determine how much profit is made after paying expenses are:

- the number of children enrolled and the tuition charged
- how much is paid for staff salaries and benefits
- the ratio of staff to children required by your state regulations which determines how much is needed for payroll
- how you control your expenses
- the presence of a continued need for child care in your area.

There are innumerable factors that would have to be considered. I believe that you can make a comfortable living by owning a day care center. Some experienced owners have told me their true net pay would be higher if they worked as a director at someone else's center because they would put in a forty-hour week and be paid for that amount of work. As an owner, you are involved each day. There is no doubt that you will be thinking about the business on your off-hours, evenings and weekends. You may have your family helping you clean, paint and maintain the general appearance of your center on Saturdays and Sundays.

If you follow the advice in this guidebook and do your homework about needs assessment, site location and compliance with the rules of all regulatory entities, your risk factor should be low. Since day care is definitely an issue of the Nineties, with anticipated growth in the next decade, the emergence of quality day care centers should be welcomed.

CAUTION:

Although it may appear to be profitable to operate a large center because of the cost-effectiveness of spreading the overhead expenses over a larger number of children or locations, I would advise you to start out on a smaller scale. Unless you have a great deal of experience in day care management, you would be wise to start on a small scale, with about twenty children. If all goes well and you still enjoy the business with the inherent rewards and disappointments, you can announce your expansion plans. To jump right in and enroll one hundred children or more is a great responsibility.

WHAT DO I NEED TO START A BUSINESS?

Call 1-800-827-5722, the Small Business Administration. They can answer your questions and help you with a wide range of subjects. They may offer a self-assessment questionnaire of your aptitude to own a business. If you score high in the areas of physical health and problem solving and if you are a risk taker, good decision maker, a people person, you will probably feel comfortable owning a business. The SBA will provide information on how to get a loan, run a new business, promote and advertise. Their workshops and publications are especially appreciated by entrepreneurs who have never started or operated a business before. The SBA is like having your own business consultant! If this phone number is not operational, call directory assistance and ask for the telephone number of the Small Business Administration in your area. Again, I urge you to search the library and bookstore for titles that offer advice about forming a business entity, selecting a logo and slogan, registering a fictitious name, applying for insurance and occupancy permits and marketing a service business.

You may require assistance in the following areas:

■ **Fictitious Name Approval**

The fictitious name is also known as DBA (doing business as) or as an assumed name. Selecting a catchy name for your center is important, but you must be sure that no other business is using the same name. When you choose a name, it should describe clearly the type of business it is. When people see the name written, they should immediately associate it with a day care business.

Register your name with the county clerk's office or the state. You will have to publish the fictitious name in a newspaper. The clerk can give you all of the specifics and a list of the acceptable newspapers in which to publish in your area. Also ask how often you have to refile to protect your selected name. Request at least three copies of this approval. Be sure to ask if any other registration is required in your area. Your lawyer or licensing representative can help you file this simple form. A small fee will be charged.

You may choose to use a name that is similar to one that is in use. This may cause confusion. Check the fictitious name registry in your state to see if your proposed name has been used. You could also check area telephone books. (You do not need to pay someone to do this for you as it is something you can easily do yourself.) Be sure that you do not infringe on someone else's logo or business slogan.

■ Bank Account

Begin a checking account and charge account in your business name. Start an organized filing system for record keeping. You must keep track of fees, charges and expenses as they're paid. Write checks or charge everything so that you have supporting documents for your expenses at tax time. You will probably need a copy of your fictitious name approval, your federal tax identification number (assigned by the IRS) and a document as to how your business is structured (sole proprietorship, partnership or corporation) when you open an account.

WHERE CAN I OBTAIN FUNDING FOR MY DAY CARE CENTER?

■ Bank Loans

Visit several banks. Be professional in all of your dealings. Dress for success! Read a few books that discuss commercial loans, business plans and banking in general. Try to at least understand some of the banking terms before you meet with the commercial loan officer.

Have a typed business plan prepared. Your librarian or accountant can show you books that give examples of how to prepare a plan. This is not absolutely necessary, but you should have at least a presentation folder prepared that explains your business concept, what you intend to do, how you intend to do it, why you think you will be successful, how much money you need to start and operate and how you plan to repay the loan. A formal business plan includes: cover page, statement of purpose, table of contents, summary of the business and financial data. An accountant or another experienced day care owner can assist you with estimates of start-up costs and operating expenses. In banking language, these are called "start-up budgets" and "operating budgets."

The loan officer will request information about your personal balance sheet such as: amount of cash in the bank, stocks or other negotiable securities, value of real estate, automobile, cash value of life insurance and other personal assets. And on the other side, how much debt do you have? Be prepared to disclose your liabilities such as loans at banks, loans to others, real estate loans, credit card and department store debts.

Banks are not in the business to give money away but will share the risk with a person with credit worthiness. You will be expected to use some of your money too. If you are refused loans by a few banks, ask the loan officer the reasons why. Then contact the SBA and inquire of their loans.

■ Grants

To learn how to apply for a grant, visit your library first. In the reference section, there are current directories that list charitable organizations, foundations and corporations that have funds to distribute. There is a way to successfully obtain a grant which includes filling out the applications carefully. Research the foundation before making application because they may only fund certain types of programs or may only accept applications at certain times of the year. If possible, call or visit the foundation office before making the application to get a feel for the process. Request a copy of their guidelines, forms and application. For more information about grants and foundations, contact:

The Foundation Center
79 Fifth Avenue, 8th floor
New York, NY 10003
212-620-4230

The Grantsmanship Center
103 S. Grand Ave.
Los Angeles, CA 90015
213-482-9860 / 1-800-421-9512

■ Private Investors

Ask local community organizations, business groups, the Chamber of Commerce, Lions Club or Parent Teacher Association if they would contribute money for a particular aspect of your business. Since you will be providing a service for the working community, they may be willing to subsidize indoor exercise mats, toys, library, a loan fund for improvements, playground equipment, tuition scholarship for a needy family, cribs for the infant room, etc. They may contribute an "in-kind" donation of their services to help you print brochures, develop a marketing plan or draw up blue-prints. Be sure to express your gratitude in writing via a letter to the editor of the local newspaper or place a commemorative plaque in a very conspicuous location in your center's lobby. This would be a good news item or photo opportunity for the newspapers too! Your center and the kind benefactor would receive valuable exposure.

■ Family and Friends

Private investors, also known as friends and family members, who believe in what you are doing and have money to lend are sources of funds. Don't forget to consider your credit union or borrowing from the cash value of your own life insurance policy. You may have a few thousand dollars that could come in handy. Check with your life insurance agent.

■ Corporations or Nursing Homes

If you are experienced in day care administration or are well connected in business, you might approach corporations about providing on-site child care. Some industries and corporations have corporate gift money available. Individuals who have successfully organized centers for employees stress that you might have to have a two-pronged approach. Since corporate decisions are not made at the personnel department level, you should address your correspondence and follow-up call to the president of the company, with a secondary letter to the personnel director. Day care centers operating in nursing homes and retirement villages are also beginning to grow in popularity. There is a book titled

Hand in Hand: A Guide to Intergenerational Programming which is available by sending $8 to: Hand in Hand, Route 2, Box 297, Monticello, MN 55362.

■ **Small Business Administration**

The SBA can assist in your efforts to locate sources of capital and funds especially if you are a woman or a member of a minority group. Contact them about your eligibility. Ask about the organization, SCORE, which is the Service Corp. Of Retired Executives. These volunteers are available to act as free consultants for any business. They are a valuable source of information and should be one of your priority contacts. Don't delay in contacting them.

■ **State Regulatory Agency**

Ask a knowledgeable state licensing representative if there are any grants, fellowships or monies set aside for centers that cater to a particular special interest group. If you qualify, you would not need private investment funds. Groups such as the United Way, Catholic Charities, Jewish Philanthropic, the League of Women Voters, Kiwanis, Rotary and the Junior League can be approached. They may contribute funds, a building, time, renovations or advice and assistance with legal, marketing and accounting issues.

■ **Civic Organizations**

Check to see if there are any civic organizations or corporations that are willing to sponsor a child or children or underwrite the cost of a project. A church may be able to donate space. A corporation that would benefit by having quality child care in close proximity might donate money, products, a building or land. Don't hesitate to ask, you might just get what you need!

The following organizations have been involved in the child care crisis in the United States. For more information and to ask about their involvement, contact:

National Council of Jewish Women
53 West 23rd Street
New York, NY 10010
212-645-4048

Kiwanis International Office
3636 Woodview Trace
Indianapolis, IN 46268-3196
800-879-4769

The Association of
Junior Leagues
660 First Avenue
New York, NY 10016
212-683-1515

Michigan 4C Association
2875 Northwind Drive, Suite 200
East Lansing, MI 48823

YWCA of the USA (Program Services)
726 Broadway
New York, NY 10003
212-614-2700

YMCA of the USA (Program Services)
101 North Wacker Drive
Chicago, IL 60606
312-977-0031

WHAT COSTS AND EXPENSES DO I NEED TO CONSIDER?

This list is just a brief overview of some expenses that you will incur in the start-up and operation of a center. These costs will probably increase regularly so build that factor into your budget and tuition planning. There are some start-up costs that are usually one-time-only costs such as large equipment purchases, utility deposits, down payments and renovation costs. In the beginning, you will also need to have extra money set aside to operate since you will probably not have full enrollment tuitions to cover all of your expenses.

ADVERTISING
postage, classified ads, display ads, direct mail for publicity efforts, outdoor sign

PRINTING
flyers, brochures, enrollment forms, stationery, business cards, policy handbooks for employees and parents, photocopying costs

OFFICE EQUIPMENT
desk, chairs, lamps, filing cabinets, bookcase, typewriter, calculator, couch, copy machine, bulletin board

OFFICE SUPPLIES
stapler, purchase order forms, bookkeeping forms, filing folders, tabs, straight pins, thumbtacks, paper clips, fasteners, paper, tape, markers, calendar, glue, keys, ruler, appointment book, gummed labels

SECURITY DEPOSITS
rent, connection charges for utilities such as telephone, gas, electricity, water, refuse and leaf collection

MAINTENANCE SUPPLIES
brooms, buckets, mops, vacuum cleaner, waste baskets, paper products, cleaning supplies, bathroom supplies, rags, dishwasher detergent, laundry detergent, sponges, dustpan, cleanser

PROFESSIONAL FEES
lawyer, accountant, insurance premiums, licensing fees, other application fees

RENOVATION EXPENSES
carpenter, electrician, plumber. (Be extremely careful in site selection. What may appear to be a perfect location may be very costly if you have to replace wiring, add partitions, erect a fence or repair a leaking roof.)

MAINTENANCE EXPENSES
grounds maintenance, snow removal, carpet cleaning, window washing, exterminator service, repair of indoor and outdoor play equipment

CLASSROOM EXPENSES
tables, chairs, cots, mats, TV, blackboard, record player

MISCELLANEOUS
toys, games, puzzles, arts and crafts supplies (buy in quantity), interest on borrowed money, cost of professional subscriptions, conferences, memberships, on-going training for staff, fire extinguishers, first-aid kit, field trip costs

Unfortunately, you must anticipate some bad debt, people who do not pay you or checks that do not clear the bank.

WHAT ARE OTHER MAJOR EXPENDITURES?

Regulations vary by locale but experienced directors have told me of large expenditures for the installation of a commercial type kitchen with three sinks, an industrial type dishwashing machine and special laundry facilities for washing sheets, diapers, smocks and other items. Separate bathrooms may be required either for adults and children, boys and girls. What type of flooring is required? Carpet, vinyl or both? Is an on-site playground required? Before you panic, check with your licensing representative for clarification of the above major expenditures. In most states, they are not required.

WHAT SHOULD I CHARGE PER WEEK?

Tuition rates vary around the country. It is hard to believe but I have heard of fees as low as $40 and as high as $190 (1993 rates). If more than one child per family is enrolled, a small discount is usually granted. Some schools charge a nominal pre-registration fee. This discourages parents from changing their plans at the last minute. If you call around to other centers—using an assumed name—you might ask for their rates. Often the director will not quote this information over the phone and you will be invited to make an appointment to visit the center.

Perhaps you have a friend with a preschooler who could help you with this "research" by visiting centers, collecting brochures, asking questions about programs, hours, policies and credentials of the staff. Your friend's report can provide valuable information in planning your center.

Your fees should be competitive and must be adequate to cover expenses for the type of day care to be offered, the hours of operation, the number of daily meals and snacks served. Fees should be collected in a business-like fashion and receipts should be given. Occasionally, fees might be waived or reduced according to hardship situations such as illness or divorce. Experienced directors have stressed not to allow families to get behind in their payments—delinquent or unpaid balances may accumulate into uncollectible debts. You may want to offer a discount on a child's enrollment, valid until a certain date before opening or in the beginning phase of advertising your business.

Several day care centers allow their parents to pay tuition using credit cards such as Mastercard or Visa. You should inquire about how to extend credit using this method of collection. Call your bank; they will probably charge you a fixed percentage of each transaction as a service charge. You could also offer a discount for those parents who pay you a month or two weeks in advance.

Remember that you will not reach full enrollment immediately. In interviewing 100 directors for this guidebook, I was told that it took at least six to nine months to reach ninety percent capacity. Also because your operating expenses will increase annually, new tuition rates will be established each year. You will want to send a letter home to the parents well in advance advising of tuition changes. Be sure to explain that you are flexible in special cases so that the hardship is not too extreme for families who need special consideration.

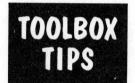

TOOLBOX TIPS

"Babies need quick responses in order to understand their world and to trust the adults who care for them. Routines build this trust. Toddlers and preschoolers feel in control of life when they routinely wash hands before meals, read stories before naps, or play outside just before going home. Life feels manageable with routines. Older children, like the younger ones, benefit from knowing the boundaries. If school age children routinely get snacks upon arrival, they know that soon they can begin their play without feeling hungry. Routines help with transition times."

Kapers For Kids
Credit: Bev Greene, Editor,
Curriculum and Craft Kits

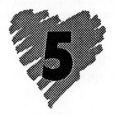

Administration

WHAT TYPES OF FORMS ARE REQUIRED?

Listed below are general ideas for forms. Because we live in a very litigious society, where people will sue when they perceive they have been wronged, you must ask a lawyer to review the wording of all forms, contracts, agreements used in your center. These are only meant to show you what I have seen other centers use, thus no liability is assumed for their use.

The state regulatory agency provides required forms. Examples are shown in the appendix of this book for my home state of Pennsylvania.

1. **Application For Day Care Service:** date of application, name of child, address, birthdate, home telephone number, business telephone number, physician's name and telephone number, any special disability, special medical, dietary or allergic conditions, health insurance information and signature of parents, persons designated to pick up child.

2. **Fee Agreement:** fee charged, number of hours included, payment schedule, services included (child care, transportation, meals, materials fee, field trip fee), arrival and departure time.

3. **Child Health Appraisal:** review of child's health history and special medical information to be filled out by physician. Includes immunization information and general developmental appraisal.

4. **Parental Consent:** this form, which includes the name of the day care facility, the child's name and written permission granted for emergency medical care, accompanies the child in the event emergency medical care is needed. In addition, it gives permission for the caregiver to administer prescription medicine (a specific list of all that can be administered and the dosage is included). A checklist for parental permission to leave the center for field trips, swimming outings, transportation by facility, etc., together with a space for the parent's signature and date for each event are also listed.

5. **Accident Report Form:** name of child, type of injury, date, time, details of accident, location, treatment provided, name of witness, signature. Consult your day care regulations for the situations that you are required to report to the licensing agency.

6. **Staff Record:** name, address, training experience, education, previous employment, health appraisal, written references, staff emergency information sheet.

7. **Fire Drill Record:** record month, day and time of each fire drill.

8. **Master Medication Log:** record date, name of child, medication and dosage administered, time, staff member who gave medicine.

9. **Field Trip Follow-up Form:** a simple way to have teacher note the location of trip, points of interest visited, reaction of group, evaluation and comments, any special problems, accidents, signature and date, etc. As a director, you want to be apprised of everything that happens both within and outside of your facility.

10. **Progress Report For Parent Conference:** the classroom teacher familiar with the child should fill out this form designed to facilitate communication with the parents. A lot of thought should be given to each item before the parent/teacher conference. Usually included is a checklist which elicits a response as to how the child reacts to being without parents all day, child-group relationships, relationship with adults, ability to share, level of participation, adaptation to day care routine, activity preferences, any signs of emotional/physical discomforts, child's social behavior, napping and meal patterns, unusual behavior noted, observation of physical health, etc. Be sure to allow time for parents to ask questions and make suggestions.

11. **Authorization To Release Information About Child:** occasionally, you may observe a child that you believe has special needs, physical or emotional. You may not contact psychological and diagnostic services on behalf of the child without written permission from the parents. A form should be designed that authorizes you to furnish pertinent information concerning the child and the family to a third party. Failure to do so could result in legal accountability.

12. **Parent Suggestions Form:** to improve services for the families, make a form available for comments. A suggestion box could be provided or the parents could discuss these issues at a parent meeting. Ask the parents for ideas for a parents discussion group. The center would arrange to have speakers from organizations address topics of interest to working parents.

13. **Volunteer Form:** should be filled out as completely as an employee application. Verify references. Require a physical examination. Obtain a criminal clearance. In addition to the usual questions, ask about special interests or training in health, art, music, dance, athletics, etc. Specify the amount of time to be volunteered and inquire as to why they feel they would make a good volunteer in a day care center. A trial period is also recommended for volunteers. Be aware of what regulations apply for volunteers caring for children in your particular state. Volunteers may be recruited at college fraternities and sororities, student teacher programs, high school home economics departments, senior citizen groups, training programs, Scouts, Foster Grandparent Programs, etc.

14. **Supply Requisition Form:** as your housekeeping, arts and crafts and snack supplies are consumed, keep informed so that you reorder before the inventory has been depleted. The form should include: date, item needed, on-hand amount, requesting teacher's name.

15. **Observation Form:** day care workers who are involved with children for long periods of time are usually able to identify some problems which may need attention. Design a form to note unusual activities such as:

temper tantrums	restlessness
hyperactivity	lethargic behavior
poor coordination	headaches, stomachaches
hearing or vision problems	rash, bruises, sores
frequent urination	restless during sleep
afraid of being alone	generally not satisfied
afraid of adults	sad disposition
afraid of strangers	moodiness

16. **Daily Infant Form:** parents like to know the daily routine of their baby. A form should provide information about: feeding schedule, quantity consumed, sleeping pattern, vomiting, fever, diaper rash, reactions to food or milk, problems or worries, and additional supplies needed from the parents such as powder, baby food, bottles, ointment, etc.

ADDITIONAL RECOMMENDED FORMS

These forms are not required, however I have found them to be useful.

1. **Checklist For Safety:** make a checklist of the possible safety hazards. At least once a week, evaluate by checking the building, indoor equipment and outdoor play area against the optimum safety list. Are doors unobstructed? Is all equipment in good repair? Are bathroom and kitchen facilities sanitary?

2. **Application For Professional Employment:** Preprinted forms can be purchased at a stationery or business supply store. Or design your own. A lawyer should approve any employment form before using it. Preprinted forms usually include lines for applicant's name, address, telephone number, health data, emergency contact information, present and previous employment information history, education completed, additional training or relevant coursework, special qualifications, reference information, etc. Some of these questions could get you in trouble legally so do your homework before selecting or designing an employee application form.

3. **Authorization Form To Contact Previous Employer:** as a reference, this form is designed so that the prospective employee authorizes you to contact past employers or references in order to pose questions about suitability for employment. Do not assume that you can contact a reference without written permission.

4. **Staff Evaluation Form:** conduct staff performance evaluations regularly. A form might show strengths and weaknesses in the following areas: punctuality, reliability, good judgement, relationships with children, parents and staff, attitude. Under personal qualities: friendliness, warmth,

sense of humor, understanding of children, tolerance, patience, flexibility, cooperation, professional attitude, etc. You are bound to think of other traits to add to the list.

There is a great book called, *Forms Kit for Directors*, available through Redleaf Press. (See address and phone number in appendix.) So that you do not have to design or type hundreds of forms for your center, you should review the suggested forms. Always check with your lawyer about use of forms. Just because they are in someone's book does not mean that they meet the current law.

TIPS ON STAFF SELECTION

How does an employer determine who to hire for a particular job? What interview techniques are most useful? How does an applicant assess desire for and satisfaction with a particular kind of job? Day care center administrators may find the following suggestions helpful in interviewing applicants for staff positions.

In a job interview, the administrator should know the questions to ask and should encourage questions of the applicant. While it is hard to determine an applicant's ability to work with children solely from an interview, the administrator can attempt to judge the applicant's attitudes toward children, discipline and new ideas. A trial period from four to eight weeks is advisable for staff members, so both administrators and employees can test their abilities in working with children and other staff members. Procedures for terminating jobs without undue strain should be set.

Finally, administrators should arrange for potential staff members to talk with other people in their field, and to share ideas about the work involved at day care centers.

WHAT ABOUT ADMINISTRATIVE PROCEDURES?

A director, the staff and the parents share the responsibility for seeing that a day care center program runs smoothly and meets the needs of the children and families. To facilitate this kind of administration, the following suggestions are presented.

1. Establish a grievance procedure, so every staff member and parent will know how and where to express complaints and can voice opinions through established channels.

2. Have frequent informal sessions to discuss problems or special conditions long before a major crisis erupts.

3. Stress open acknowledgment of, and sensitive awareness to, possible difficulties when there are ethnic differences between staff and children.

4. Develop good communication between staff and parents. Parents should be included, whenever possible, in the decision-making processes.

5. Be responsive to each individual staff member as a human being, with a life both inside and outside the center.

6. Do not allow the center to be exclusively child-centered, although the primary staff function is care of children. Children need to experience the world of adults as it touches their lives, in order to learn their place in that world.

7. Assign parents working as staff members to a room or section other than that where their own children are placed. It is difficult for both child and parent to develop new ways of relating to each other, and it is unfair to other children if one is singled out for special attention and care.

8. Tell staff members when they are succeeding and when they need to re-evaluate their behavior as staff members.

9. Consider the need for staff counseling at all levels. A counselor who helps with personal and professional problems is important in this kind of personally exhaustive work.

10. For a smoothly functioning staff, be willing to adapt to the needs of both adults and children. Many employees will be women with their own families. Often, complicated day care arrangements must be made to free them to work.

11. Remember that staff members grow and change. Continuing to treat someone as a trainee long after he/she is a fully-functioning member of the staff may lead to dissatisfaction and disappointment.

12. Turnover may be a major problem, and to minimize this, eliminate some of the most frequently disturbing situations leading to resignations, such as long hours, limited opportunities for advancement, lack of privacy, uneasy relations with other staff members, difficult children to care for without extra support, high demands on the stamina and physical energy of the staff, and low salaries.

13. Clarify work arrangements. Don't assume that a job description, once given, is completely absorbed and understood.

14. Provide opportunities for constant learning and outside stimulation. It is all too easy to become bored by working exclusively with infants and young children all day. To prevent this, staff members might occasionally exchange duties. Also arrangements could be made for staff to attend special meetings and conferences, observe in other centers, and have discussions with other staff members about children and on-the-job problems. Outside speakers can be invited to talk at staff meetings and abundant, interesting reading material can be made available.

WHAT IS THE STAFF-CHILD RATIO?

To guarantee optimal development of infants and young children in group care, a low ratio of children to caregivers is preferable. High quality of a few will not make up for an insufficient number of caregivers. But neither will a large number of caregivers substitute for quality care. Caregivers who must supervise a large number of children may neglect certain children and become exhausted. States differ in their licensing requirements regarding ratios.

WHAT ARE SOME CHARACTERISTICS OF GOOD CAREGIVERS?

Obviously, no one person will have all the qualities described here. Initially, however, a caregiver should already have some of these characteristics; others may be acquired through training and experience. In general, the following qualities are important for a good caregiver.

THE CAREGIVER SHOULD:

■ be patient and warm toward children. This warmth is the basic ingredient in the caregiver-child relationship. Only with patience can the child be helped to develop and the caregiver survive the strains of this type of work.

■ like children, be able to give personally to them and receive satisfaction from what they have to offer. They must be able to appreciate the baby as an individual, since this is vital to the baby's growing self-acceptance. A caregiver also needs to have a sense of humor.

■ understand that children need more than simple physical care. They should have some knowledge of the practical care of children and be willing and able to learn from other people.

■ be able to adjust to various situations, understand feelings and help children to handle fear, sadness and anger, as well as to experience love, joy and satisfaction.

■ be in good health. Since children possess abundant energy, the caregiver must be energetic and imaginative in order to teach and discipline them.

■ be aware of the importance of controlling undesirable behavior, but must not be punitive or given to outbursts of anger.

■ show initiative and resourcefulness in working with children and be able to adapt the program to meet their individual needs and preferences.

■ be acquainted with, accept and appreciate the children's cultures, customs and languages if they are different from their own. Helping the child develop a sense of pride in their own uniqueness is vital.

■ respect the child and their parents, regardless of their backgrounds or particular circumstances, thus helping the child learn to respect himself. The caregivers own self-respect will aid in imparting this quality to others.

■ be able to work with other adults and get along with the other staff members in order to provide a harmonious atmosphere at the center.

■ have a positive interest in learning, understand the importance and variety of learning needs in a young child, and be responsive to the child's attempt at learning in all spheres.

SHOULD I USE VOLUNTEERS AS STAFF IN THE DAY CARE CENTER?

The use of volunteers in a day care center is a debatable topic. Their interest in children and their help can add to the program. However, volunteers should not work directly with children unless they show a great aptitude for this kind of work and agree to accept supervision. A volunteer who appears on some days and not on others may destroy the continuity of care for children and the morale of other staff members. Therefore, volunteers should be required to commit themselves to a definite schedule of service, although their schedules may be more flexible than those of the regular staff. In this way, the volunteers become regular, contributing and necessary members of the day care staff.

(Source for *Tips on Staff Selection* section: US Dept. of HEW, Publication 0HD5-78-31056)

ADVERTISING & PROMOTION

HOW CAN I PUBLICIZE MY BUSINESS?

There are many ways to advertise. The key thing that you must consider is—what sets your business apart from the other day care centers, down the street, in the next town or next to yours in the telephone book? Your stationery, business cards, logo, signs and all communication convey your image to the community. Become involved in the community by volunteering for charitable events, co-sponsoring affairs and socializing with people in the business community. Fellow business people will refer customers to you.

Make sure that the following agencies and organizations know of your child care center. Send flyers, an announcement or make an in-person visit to the local resource and referral agency, YWCAs, YMCAs, YWHAs, YMHAs, churches and synagogues, parent support groups. Send information to parent newsletters and newspapers. Notify the state licensing office and civic organizations such as the National Council of Jewish Women, the National Organization for Women, the Junior League, the Business and Professional Women Association and the United Way. Offer your services to speak at a meeting about a day-care related topic such as:

Is day care good for children?
Finding good child care
Current child care legislation
How to use the Federal Child Care Tax Credit

Advertising in the newspaper and phone book can be expensive. Some ideas that are less costly but effective are:

1. Obtain the names and addresses of the local newspapers. Send a press release. A press release is an announcement of some aspect of your business. Books in the library under "Public Relations" or "Publicity" will show you the precise format for writing a release that will have a good chance of appearing in the paper. A press release is just a short article about your business written in the third person. It must be written like a

news story stating who, what, where, when and why. It must not appear that you are asking for free advertising (publicity) although that is precisely your intention. Review the style of most articles in your local paper that pertain to church bazaars, school events, town meetings, pet shows, etc. They are written by the organization and are a great way of obtaining free publicity. You must publicize your own business on a regular basis. At least four times a year, stage some newsworthy event and send out press releases or call the newspaper with the details and see if they'll send a reporter and photographer out to your center.

2. Call the local "newsroom" or "city desk" of the newspaper and tell them that you are opening a new business in the area. They may want to do a "feature story" about you or some interesting aspect of the business. Try to think of an "angle" or "hook" or an unusual twist that makes your center sound special.

3. If you know of freelance newspaper reporters, give them a call. They may want to write a story (complete with pictures). They would query the newspaper with the idea and if interested the freelance writer would do the story and be paid by the newspaper. Be sure to make it sound like news, not asking for free publicity.

4. Have a "grand opening party" to coincide with registration so that prospective customers may tour your facility. Parents can meet you and your teachers and aides. A cheerfully decorated center and a safe outdoor play area can help make "the sale." Be sure to be extremely organized, enthusiastic, courteous and professional in the operation of your business. Be creative. Hire a clown to give out lollipops and balloons, offer pony rides, or pay a musician to play children's songs on an accordion, piano or banjo. You can't be shy when it comes to marketing your business. Don't forget to call the local TV news stations and the newspaper to tell them about the event. You want to generate interest and goodwill in the community.

5. Occasionally, throughout the year, hold some social or special event. Be sure to call reporters and send press releases to provide information about your puppet performance, parade, baby contest, children's used clothing exchange, family movie night, magic show, square dance, Fun Fair, Easter Egg Hunt, Breakfast with Santa, pony rides, ballet recital, child safety program, graduation ceremony, other holiday celebrations, penny auction, etc. Serve light refreshments. (This is a good public relations strategy.)

6. Contact personnel departments, colleges, pediatricians, school districts, real estate firms, civic organizations, etc., and tell them of your new business. Send them a professional looking letter or flyer announcing your service (one page only). Since this is a reflection on you, be sure to have someone proofread it for spelling, grammar and general appearance. You only get one chance to make a good first impression. You will have to print brochures, flyers and business cards. You may find a local independent printer who is less expensive than a stationery store or franchise printer. (Be sure to look at samples of the work before ordering.)

7. Consider it "news" and call reporters if you decide to add any new services: special needs child day care, full day kindergarten, senior citizen day care, drop-in babysitting, weekend and evening child care, holiday or summer care, handicapped care, twenty-four hour care, or if you decide to offer transportation services.

8. If a parent has volunteered to demonstrate some special skill or talent at your center, let the media know about it. Small local newspapers are anxious to list these types of events in their calendar of events. How about a special one-hour seminar explaining the Child Care Tax Credit, if applicable?

9. One center prepared recorded messages that changed weekly on a separate phone number. The three-minute message discussed a topic of interest to parents. Each week, the newspaper printed the topic, phone number and name of the center (good free advertising and great public relations).

10. Design a colorful flyer. Make copies. Modify the flyer to suit your program and your credentials. Make a pocket out of construction paper or a "take one box" to hold your flyers. Decorate the construction paper with cut-outs from magazine pictures of mothers, children, etc. Post on bulletin boards in supermarkets, community centers, hair salons, libraries, churches, pediatrician offices, laundromats and wherever parents congregate. Don't forget about putting flyers on car windshields in shopping center parking lots. You can hire and supervise some older kids to help you with this one.

11. If your newspaper has inexpensive advertising rates, you may be successful by placing an ad in the classified or display ad section. People usually have to see something repeated about five times to be effective, so advertising in a newspaper can't just be done on a one-time basis. Advertise continuously in one way or another. Be sure to have your center listed by any free referral services for child care. Ask your licensing bureau for the names of the child care resource and referral services in your area.

12. Many day care centers have said that word of mouth has been their best form of advertisement—the percentage of new clients enrolled is greatest when satisfied parents spread the good word. Ask each parent how they heard of your center. After enrollment, send them a thank-you note explaining your desire to make it a very pleasant experience for their family.

13. Hold a Parents Night Out. This could be a time when you offer discussion periods or lectures on career/day care related topics such as: child abuse, stress, child rearing issues, managing work and family, positive parenting techniques, behavior modification, etc.

14. Place an ad in the Yellow Pages. Look in several out-of-town phone books to see how other centers advertise their business.

15. Make sure that your outside sign and the exterior of your facility is attractive, eye-catching and neat.

16. Tell everyone that you know about your business (friends, relatives, neighbors, acquaintances, former co-workers).

WHAT ELSE CAN I DO FOR PROMOTION?

In an art supply or book store, you will find books called "Clip Art" or "Dover Art." These are books filled with logos (pictures) which are not usually covered by copyright legislation (so you are able to use these cute pictures on your stationery, brochures, business cards, etc.).

Contact local radio and talk shows and ask to be a guest. Believe it or not, the smaller ones in your area will probably schedule you immediately! You could offer to talk about any day care related topic such as "What Parents Should Look For In Quality Centers." Of course, this is great exposure for your center and a fun experience for you.

Finally, even the large television stations have "slow news" days. Our center was featured on all three of the major networks. There really was nothing special, but roving reporters covered it at different times and we received excellent recommendations. One comical situation was right after we opened. The enrollment was 5 children and two staff members. The center was beautifully decorated and equipped, however we were just starting out...so the center was not near capacity. A TV news reporter called and said that the mini-camera van was in the area covering another major event and they had noticed our "Grand Opening" sign. They were on their way to pay us a visit. Since I only had a half hour before they would arrive, I quickly ran to the local supermarket and the library and told all mothers with small children that if they wanted their children on the evening news to quickly comb their hair, wash their faces and like the "Pied Piper," follow me. By the time the TV reporter arrived, we had a center filled with beautiful children playfully using all of the equipment and having a wonderful time. A staged performance? Yes! Successful exposure, without a doubt!

Another promotional attempt was when we rented two "attention-getting" costumes from a costume center. An eight-foot Sesame Street Big Bird look-a-like and a seven-foot dalmatian were hard to ignore. It's hard to believe that we did this, but it did have the desired effect. My associate and I donned the extremely heavy and hot costumes and stood on a major highway causing everyone to look twice. Armed with hundreds of flyers and balloons with our center's name, we passed out our promotional pieces. We even walked around several industrial complexes. Of course, we prayed that no one would even think it was us. Our hope was that people would think that we had hired high school freshmen for this job. Newspaper photographers thought it was a little odd so they snapped pictures which appeared in the evening newspaper along with our day care center's name. Just another means of publicity and exposure but it was worth the $80 costume rental fee.

When people see "Sitting Service," they may approach you with another care-giving need other than for children. One very nice man stopped in and asked if we might be able to help him with "bird sitting" for his two zebra finches. He had to go to California for two weeks and had no one to feed them. He thought, and we foolishly agreed, that the birds in their decorative cages would be interesting for the children. He came in the next week and attached hooks for the cages and proudly told us of all of the precious moments of joy he experienced raising his two rare "babies." You guessed it! Both of them died during his absence. We fed them, talked to them, sang to them and provided excellent aviary care. Apparently they did not like the air conditioning. After worrying needlessly while we waited for the "proud papa" to return, we were surprised to find out he wasn't at all upset. Moral of story: make child care your specialty! "No bird watching" should be a part of your policy.

WHEN IS THE BEST TIME TO OPEN?

Summers are generally a slower period and enrollment is usually down. Many people are on vacation and/or are reluctant to make day care changes. A "grand opening" in September, with registration accepted in the summer may be okay. Also, January is a good time—coinciding with the school semester. A summer camp for school-age children may be organized to fill in for the absence of tuition payments from your regular students.

ADVICE FROM THE EXPERTS

TIPS FROM "EXPERIENCED DIRECTORS"

During research for this chapter, many day care directors were asked for their input. Their sage advice follows.

GETTING STARTED

1. Double the time that you think will be required to open a day care center. Some of the delays in opening will be beyond your control since there may be confusion among the many regulatory agencies. Plan to be in the center at least a month before opening to ensure that everything is in place and that all necessary documents have been obtained and posted.

2. Enroll in courses at adult evening schools to study Small Business Management or Entrepreneurship, so that you are familiar with tax liability, insurance issues, recordkeeping, legal issues, incorporation, marketing, public relations, etc. In addition to knowledge about day care, to be successful, you must also have sound business, financial and management skills.

3. Visit other day care centers. Of course, due to the threat of friendly and non-friendly competition, many local directors will not be too anxious to help you out so visit centers in other nearby cities. Observe their programs. After you leave, jot down your impressions—positive and negative. If possible, try to obtain a copy of their "Parent Handbook" as a

guide for planning your own (see Number 56). Call community colleges that have day care centers. Make an appointment to observe their operation. They would be more amenable to your visit than a private center. Start a file on day care. Study newspapers and magazines to see how people advertise. Copy the techniques that are used to attract attention. Clip the following about day care related subjects: newspaper articles about other centers, display ads describing programs, classified ads advertising for staff, photographs of centers. Notice their specialties and the "buzz words" that are used to describe the center. Note the name of the person who writes the articles related to your area of interest and set up a meeting. Look for a feature writer in either the Business or Living section.

4. Call 800-424-2460 (National Association for the Education of Young Children) and ask for the telephone number of the NAEYC chapter in your city. Attend their meetings as a means of networking. Experienced day care directors and teachers will share their expertise about provider salaries and benefits, leadership in Early Childhood Programs, time management, time-savers, handling staff conflicts and grievances, pending legislation, eligible programs for state-licensed centers, etc., if you are a member of this excellent association. Be sure to read *Young Children*, a publication of NAEYC. Also join other professional business associations. Offer to speak to community groups about issues related to day care. It is a good public relations strategy and an excellent way to promote your center.

5. Contact the licensing bureau in your state to clarify the requirements if you plan to be affiliated with a church, school or synagogue. Are there any special requirements when requesting church status?

6. A successful day care business usually depends on an owner-operated facility. Turning the reins of management over to a manager is risky. No one cares about the success as much as you do. (In my experience I have seen several cases where a trusted employee was tempted by the collection of cash and loose recordkeeping. The absentee owners lost a substantial amount of money before the loopholes were discovered.) As a director, you should be involved with the teachers and children. "Pop in" regularly to each classroom and observe. Unless you keep a watchful eye on every aspect of the care offered in your center, you might not be aware of what is really going on.

7. Network with local day care associations so you are plugged into problems, legislative issues and new resources. Before opening a day care center, consider being a volunteer in an existing center to observe first-hand daily routines, procedures, classroom environment, practices and problems.

8. Many people are just "shopping" by calling every center in the phone book. Rather than give too much information over the phone, take their name and phone number and set up a time for them to visit your center. After greeting the parent and child warmly, take them on a tour and follow up with an information package that includes: brochure, fee

schedule, general policies and procedures, etc. Be sure to give the parent plenty of time to ask questions.

9. Don't overlook the possibility of using your center during "off hours" for evening and weekend babysitting. Another center offers dinners to go and on-site haircuts as a convenience for parents. The catering service that prepares the lunches for the children takes weekly orders, payable in advance, for dinners that the parents can take home ($5 per adult and $3 per child).

10. As the owner, your enthusiasm will be contagious. Don't remain aloof from staff and children. I can't emphasize enough how important it is for you to be involved. (Don't hide in your office with administrative details.)

11. Although infant day care is in demand, state regulations require a high adult to infant staff ratio. Keep this in mind when planning staff needs and tuition charged for infant day care.

12. Imagine yourself being a child in a day care center! Remind your staff to do the same. From this vantage point you will be able to give the children the best care!

13. Don't be discouraged. It takes some time to reach full enrollment. Marketing your center is an ongoing project. Keep a supply of flyers handy at all times. Post at employment offices, laundromats, libraries, schools, personnel offices of businesses and industries, hospitals, universities, churches, etc. Let local radio and television shows know that you are available for interviews. They will introduce you as an expert in day care and as the owner of a center. Keep repeating the ideas in the publicity section of this book.

14. If there are regulations that are difficult or impossible to comply with, ask the licensing representative if you can apply for a waiver.

15. Supplies are expensive. Don't hesitate to send memos home occasionally asking parents to save styrofoam meat trays, computer paper or other things that their place of employment may be discarding.

16. Contact vocational technical schools and senior centers to help build special projects or to help with printing. Of course, make sure that the equipment is built to your exact safety standards because you are ultimately liable for everything that happens in your center. Vo-tech students may make signs, erect a fence, print flyers, business cards, newsletters and brochures, paint a wall mural, silk screen T-shirts for the kids with the center's name and logo, etc.

17. Don't overlook buying used equipment. Check the Sunday newspaper for auctions of office furniture, paper products, general supplies, refrigerated dispensers, janitorial supplies, day-to-day office

supplies and food preparation equipment. Many businesses fold and are anxious to recoup some of their money by selling their assets.

18. Be sure to do everything "first class." First impressions are lasting! Your facility should be clean and uncluttered. Your staff should be warm and loving. Your brochures and signs should all be professionally and attractively printed. Transportation vehicles should be clean and safe.

19. Have a "First Anniversary" party of your day care center to celebrate (show off) the facility, creative art projects, staff, bulletin boards, newly decorated van, new one-way observation window for parents to observe, scrapbook of photos taken at the zoo or playground, etc.

20. Fundraisers could be the sale of T-shirts, candy, baked goods, etc. Consider having a flea market or craft fair and offering exhibit tables for rent. Present your center in the best possible light.

LOCATION AND LEASING

21. The first or ground level is the most desirable location for a day care program in terms of convenience and safety. You must consider additional features when using a basement, second or third floor for a center for young children. Special considerations regarding heat, ventilation and lighting are important.

22. Be clear about the amount of playground space and indoor space required for each child. You may not need to have your own playground if there is a playground located in close proximity. Check the regulations. Write or call the U.S. Consumer Product Safety Commission, Office of the Secretary, Washington, D.C. 20207 (800-638-2772), for a booklet detailing general guidelines for new and existing playgrounds.

23. Make sure zoning rulings allow you to place a sign in front of your facility. What size and type is permitted? Are there zoning restrictions regarding traffic patterns or parking arrangements?

24. Don't underestimate problems which are associated with asbestos in a building, lead paint, fire alarms, noise levels which may not be acceptable to neighbors and parking problems.

25. Before making the decision to open a corporate day care center, conduct a thorough needs assessment survey. Employees may initially say that they think it is a great idea but in reality would not use it if available.

26. Beware of long term leases or leases that are not advantageous to you. Landlord and tenant must agree in writing about the proposed use of the facility: (1) Are you permitted to add on to expand? (2) Are there any limitations to the site's use? (3) How will you mediate disputes? (4) Will you be allowed to use outdoor space for a playground? (5) Can you erect a fence? (6) Can you use space after normal day care hours for meetings or

activities and events? (7) Agree on rental fee and time availability of building. (8) Be sure that all plumbing and sewer systems are operable. (9) Decide who will be responsible for repairs, maintenance, snow removal, lawn care, etc.

27. Before signing a lease or purchase agreement, determine a realistic estimate for the costs of remodeling, renovating, construction, alterations, repairing. How about upkeep for the kitchen, bathroom, playroom, parking lot and laundry room? Would you have to add storage closets, shelves, carpeting, linoleum, additional lighting, improved ventilation, fire escapes, new asphalt for the parking lot and driveway, new heater, electrical wiring, bathroom fan or window or new roof? In many states, fire safety laws dictate that all doors must open outward and be equipped with panic hardware. Are screens in place on each window? Exposed radiators will probably need to be enclosed for safety.

BUDGETS AND EXPENSES

28. Don't forget to consider replacement costs and utility rate increases when planning your budget. Equipment wears out, supplies are consumed and phone, electric and water costs do not remain constant.

29. Transportation costs include vehicles' purchase or rental price, insurance premiums, inspections, maintenance, oil, gas, etc. Be sure all of this is considered when setting your fees.

30. Occasionally, you will have uncollectible fees (people withdraw children without notice or payment). It is recommended to have parents pay a week in advance and notify you two weeks in advance of plans for withdrawal.

31. Keep expenses under control! It is tempting to buy fancy equipment but remember that most businesses fail due to excessive spending and poor recordkeeping.

32. You can recruit handymen to help with basic repairs, painting and fix-up. Contact college students, retired people or the city youth program. Place ads in local newspapers. Check references and agree on fees charged for service. Workmen should only be present on weekends or after hours. No work should be done while the children are in the building. You could also ask parents if they are able to recommend competent and dependable workers. High schools, community colleges, vocational schools and universities may have a pool of potential helpers for special projects.

EMPLOYEE REQUIREMENTS

33. Be clear about the level of education required to be a director, teacher or owner of a center. Are you sure that you qualify? What qualifications are required of: administrator, group supervisor, aides, infant

nursery supervisor, assistant director, food service worker, cook or vehicle driver for transportation?

34. Be sure that staff members know their roles, school philosophy and responsibilities. (Remember that your staff can make or break the reputation and ultimate success of your business.) Be clear about the staff following your personal safety standards (and the state regulations) and approved methods of discipline. Developing an employee handbook to help new hires and substitutes is a good idea (see Number 40). Make sure that your staff projects your image for a professional center. Do they dress neatly and behave appropriately with parents and children? Are they friendly and positive? Do they treat the children with respect and affection?

35. Keep aware of morale and motivation problems. Be good to your staff. Help them to keep up their enthusiasm and avoid burnout. Low salaries and the absence of benefits are the main reasons for quick turnover of day care employees.

36. Have a trial period for new staff members.

37. Before hiring staff, study the general requirements for age of staff and volunteers. Be sure to have on file health appraisals, state police clearance, child abuse clearance, written references and whatever paperwork is required before the date of hire.

38. Be sure to have a list of competent and approved substitutes. Make certain that they meet minimum age requirements and that they have a valid criminal/fingerprint clearance as determined by your state's regulations.

39. Contact the Early Childhood department of local colleges for substitute workers, teachers or just advice on quality early childhood programs. Is there an early childhood specialist that could visit your center and present information on the do's and don'ts of discipline? Some traits of competent staff workers are friendliness, high energy level, good judgement, the ability to instill confidence with the parents, well-adjusted and a love for children. Check all references thoroughly.

40. Develop an employee handbook which details hiring policies, salary range, benefits, training opportunities, absence policies, holidays, vacation, expectations in working with children and parents, classroom and playground rules, health and safety procedures, etc. Review this with each prospective employee and discuss frequently at staff meetings so that you are aware of any "gripes." You want to keep your employees satisfied, so it is best to listen to their suggestions.

41. You may want to recruit volunteers from community colleges, local universities and nursing schools. Pediatric nursing students may have to study the "well child." It is advisable to have a definite plan of activities

for them to follow. Be sure that volunteers meet the qualifications of your state licensing bureau and are covered by the fine print of your insurance policy. Since this practice teaching may be considered as an internship or student teaching, be sure to give them responsible tasks and monitor their progress so you can report back to their instructors.

42. Provide money for staff training at workshops, conferences and for renting movies on child development and day care issues. Let your staff know that you are interested in furthering their professional development. Subscribe to early childhood publications such as *Child Care Information Exchange, Pre-K Today, Child Care News* and *Young Children.* Contact the American Academy of Pediatrics. They maintain a registry of health professionals who are willing to give advice on early childhood programs. Ask a nutritionist or pediatric specialist to provide information on healthy snacks, easy-to-prepare meals, child safety topics, fluoride, dental health and handwashing procedures.

43. Investigate which state agencies or community resource groups can provide federal subsidies and free staff training on safety and nutrition. Inquire about training available for preschool staff regarding first-aid procedures, positive discipline, child safety, behavior modification, etc. Ask your state licensing bureau representative to help you access further resource information.

44. Your staff should be trained in emergency First Aid procedures. Ongoing staff training in all areas contributes to the success and professionalism of your center. Studies have shown that high quality day care centers make ongoing staff training a priority. Contact the Child Care Employee Project for information on the impact of the quality of care relative to child care provider training and support. Their National Child Care Staffing Study explored how teachers and their working conditions affected the caliber of center-based child care (510-653-9889).

HEALTH AND SAFETY

45. Have a small "sick room" with a comfortable bed for children who are waiting for a parent to pick them up. Children should be inspected each morning as a health check. Conjunctivitis (Pink Eye) and head lice are two nuisances that are highly contagious. If you determine a child is sick, he should not be admitted.

46. Establish a working relationship with a local pediatrician to be "on call."

47. Many day care centers require disposable diapers to help provide safe and sanitary changing and play areas. A report issued by the nation's leading pediatric and public health organizations, the American Academy of Pediatrics and the American Public Health Association, recognizes the benefit of disposable diapers in day care. Check for your state's standards on diapering procedures. Disposable diapers are superior to cloth in

helping keep skin dry because the absorbent gelling material locks moisture away from the babies' skin. Modern disposable diapers help prevent leakage of urine and minimize fecal contamination of children, caregivers, environmental surfaces and objects in day care settings. According to a 1990 Gallup Survey, four out of five parents who use disposables do so largely for health reasons.

48. Find out the telephone number of the Child Abuse Hotline in your state and report abuse if you suspect that a child is being harmed or neglected.

49. Keep an accident report log that describes the nature of the injury, date, time, treatment provided and details of the laceration, burn, fall, etc. Report to your licensing bureau per your regulations.

50. Contact the U.S. Consumer Product Safety Commission for safety alerts or recalls on toys, products and playground equipment. Ask for a list of agencies that provide free or low-cost educational materials such as brochures and booklets. I was surprised by the statistic of the number of children that drowned in toilets, bathtubs, five-gallon buckets, diaper pails and bathtub supporting rings. Do not leave even a few inches of liquid in a bucket after use. Unattended children could topple forward and drown because they can not lift themselves back out.

51. The American Red Cross offers training, usually for a fee. However, there are grants/funds available for child care professionals that reduce the fee to just a few dollars per individual. Contact your local chapter of the American Academy of Pediatrics or the American Red Cross for information.

PROGRAM DEVELOPMENT

52. Is private academic school registration required in your state? If so, what additional educational requirements must be met to advertise your program as a nursery school or kindergarten? This may be under the domain of your state's Department of Education. Contact your regional day care office for information about all programs related to the care of children.

53. Learn of the resources in your state that may apply to children who have special needs.

54. When enrollment has reached capacity or if you are unable to help a parent with their child care needs, be extremely helpful anyway. This parent will tell others how cordial you were. This is good for future business and a credit to your reputation.

55. Must hot meals be served? What special food/kitchen equipment is required? Can kitchen staff be a teacher or must you hire a cook and nutritionist to prepare food? Are you permitted to use a microwave? Do

you need a commercial size refrigerator to store the children's lunches? How many kitchen sinks are required? Government agencies such as the USDA and trade groups such as the American Dietetic Association and the American School Food Service Organization work with schools to improve the nutritional quality of food served to children. Contact them for food guidelines.

RELATIONS WITH PARENTS

56. Develop a parent handbook so that sensitive communication with parents is easily facilitated. It should include: school calendar, sick policy, fee payment schedule, payment of late fees, arrival and dismissal procedures, parent contract, field trip explanation, extra clothes needed, etc. One unhappy parent who feels that they were wronged or misunderstood is capable of causing a great deal of damage to your reputation.

57. "Perception" is important. How parents perceive you, your staff, your facility and your treatment and attitude towards children are critical. Do everything that you can to make sure that your center and staff are impressive. Train your staff to maintain eye contact and extend warmth to parents and children alike.

58. Smile and create a warm welcome for the parent and the child upon arrival. If possible, the owner should be there throughout the day. Parents like to see that continuity.

59. Have a bulletin board available for parents to list carpool arrangements, to exchange services and ideas, sell used items, etc. Some system for sharing daily happenings with the parents should be implemented. Some centers send a calendar of events home each month to keep parents apprised of special events such as field trips, parents night, etc. How about a small library for parents to share books about raising children?

60. A parent newsletter could be used to offer helpful hints on child care and early childhood development, to inform parents of special art projects, parties, words to songs and learning activities so they can reinforce what is being introduced at the center. Also use the newsletter as a means to inform parents of how they can become more involved with the program.

61. Perhaps parents can trade reduced fees for assisting with repairs, sewing, landscaping, reading stories, typing, help with fundraising activities, offering parent workshops in a field that would interest other parents, etc.

62. Explain to the parents the importance of not rushing the children in the morning at drop-off or in the evening at pick-up time.

63. Children can feel depressed when home life is in turmoil. Divorce, death, sickness, family fighting or a parent away on a business trip can be very unsettling to children. Staff must be trained to be aware of changes in behavior and temperament. Ask the parents to let you know about anything that may make the child anxious so that your staff can offer extra understanding and warmth.

HOW WILL PARENTS EVALUATE YOUR CENTER?

Since day care is a very hot topic, many magazines have published articles with a checklist for comparison shopping for day care service included. Parents will probably evaluate your center and your ability to provide care by using these checklists and questions such as listed below.

1. Is the center's license current? Where is it posted?

2. What would you do if my child became ill? Is there an isolation area? Would you notify me right away? How is an emergency procedure handled?

3. Can parents visit their child during lunch hour? Are parental visits encouraged? Can parents drop in unexpectedly?

4. Would my child feel comfortable here? Is the center child- oriented? Are the children touched patiently, lovingly, gently, affectionately?

5. Do the building and playground appear safe for children? Is the center adequately staffed? Do you believe the staff can effectively supervise the children?

6. Are the rooms bright, attractive, uncluttered and well organized?

7. What is the weekly menu? What types of snacks and drinks are provided? Are meal plans posted? Are meals nutritious?

8. Is the outdoor play equipment clean and safe?

9. Are inside toys age-appropriate and in good repair?

10. Do you like the caregivers? Are they warm, open, sensitive, flexible and loving? Do they communicate with children in their "own language?" Can you establish a friendly relationship with the staff?

11. What is the philosophy of the center? Does the staff understand what curriculum they employ? Are there interesting bulletin boards and art learning projects on display?

12. Would you feel at ease discussing your concerns? Would the staff be willing to accept constructive evaluation from parents? Will the center honor your individual requests?

13. What are the discipline procedures? Is time-out used rather than spanking, shaming or yelling? What are napping procedures? Do the children appear well-rested?

14. What are diaper changing procedures? Is the diaper area disinfected after each child with a product such as LYSOL? Are you satisfied with the toilet facilities? Is the center sanitary? Do the children look clean and healthy?

15. Is there a shady area to play so children are protected from intense rays of the sun? (Sliding boards and other metal equipment may be too hot to use in the summer.)

16. Are there learning activities for each age group? Do they understand the importance of providing a wide variety of experiences for young children?

17. How does the center celebrate holidays, birthdays, etc? Is the staff understanding of cultural and ethnic differences?

18. What types of academic training do the teachers have? Do they have some in-service training in child care, child development or early childhood education? Is there ongoing training or seminar attendance sponsored by a child care organization?

19. Are seat belts/car seats provided for field trips?

20. Do the children look happy? Is there a healthy noise level at the center?

21. Do you understand the center's policies on vacation days, withdrawal procedures, payment of fees, late charges? Are the fees comparable with other centers in the area?

22. Will the schedule meet the needs of your child?

23. How will the staff communicate with you about your child's day? Will they have time to chat each day? An evening phone call? Progress reports? Will a written memo be provided? Are home visits scheduled?

24. Will there be "open houses" and conferences scheduled regularly?

25. Can parents volunteer to go on field trips or help out with special events?

26. Are the exits from the classrooms and building unobstructed for easy escape in an emergency?

27. Can they provide you with references of parents whose children currently attend the center?

28. Do they closely supervise the infants and give appropriate supervision and independence to other children?

29. Have all of the caregivers had a physical examination in order to work in the center?

TOOLBOX TIPS

Problems with Parents' Payments?

• *Begin by setting policies that clearly state your fees and due dates. Require parents to pay a nonrefundable deposit based on your notice period.*

• *Include a policy that says care will not be provided if the payments are overdue, and stick to it! If they forget the checkbook again, have them take the child with them to go get it.*

• *Require cash payments, if necessary.*

Kaleidoscope, Kapers for Kids
Credit: Bev Greene,
Curriculum Director

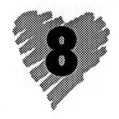

EDUCATIONAL CURRICULUM GUIDANCE

THE EDUCATION PLAN SHOULD INDICATE:

1. How the Education Program will provide children with a learning environment and varied experiences appropriate to their age and stage of development which will help them develop: socially, intellectually, physically, emotionally.

2. How the Education Program will integrate the educational aspects of the various components in the daily program of activities.

3. How the Education Program will involve parents in educational activities to enhance their role as the principal influence on the child's education and development.

4. How the Education Program will assist parents to increase knowledge, understanding skills and experience in child growth and development.

5. How the Education Program will identify and reinforce experiences which occur in the home that parents can utilize as educational activities for their children. The plan should be accompanied by brief descriptive information regarding: geographical setting, physical setting (available facilities), populations to be served (ethnicity, race, language, age, prevalence of handicapping conditions, health factors, family situations), education staff (staffing patterns, experience, training), volunteers, community resources, program philosophy/curriculum approach, assessment procedures (individual child, total program).

HOW TO ENHANCE CHILDREN'S UNDERSTANDING OF SELVES

The following suggestions may be useful beginning steps: encourage awareness of self through the use of full-length mirrors, photos and drawings of child and family, tape recordings of voices, etc.

HOW TO GIVE CHILDREN OPPORTUNITIES FOR SUCCESS

Here are some examples:

1. Make sure that activities are suited to the developmental level of each child.

2. Allow the child to do as much for himself as he can.

3. Help the child learn "self-help" skills (pouring milk, putting on coat).

4. Recognize and praise honest effort and not just results.

5. Support efforts and intervene when helpful to the child.

6. Help the child accept failure without defeat ("I will help you try again.").

7. Help the child learn to wait ("You will have a turn in five minutes.").

8. Break tasks down into manageable parts so that children can see how much progress they are making.

HOW TO PROVIDE AN ENVIRONMENT OF ACCEPTANCE

This can be accomplished by adult behavior such as:

1. Showing respect for each child.

2. Listening and responding to children.

3. Showing affection and personal regard (greeting by name, one-to-one contact).

4. Giving attention to what the child considers important (looking at a block structure, locating a lost mitten).

5. Expressing appreciation, recognizing effort and accomplishments of each child, following through on promises.

6. Respecting and protecting individual rights and personal belongings (a "cubby" or box for storage, name printed on work in large, clear letters).

7. Acknowledging and accepting unique qualities of each child.

8. Avoiding situations which stereotype sex roles or racial-ethnic backgrounds.

9. Providing ample opportunity for each child to experience success, to earn praise, to develop an "I can," "Let me try," attitude.

10. Accepting each child's language, whether it be standard English, a dialect or a foreign language, and fostering the child's comfort in using the primary language.

11. Providing opportunities to talk about feelings, to share responsibilities, to share humor.

HOW TO DEVELOP INTELLECTUAL SKILLS

Intellectual skills can be enhanced by providing a learning climate in which staff may guide children to foster cognitive functioning (i.e., understanding, reasoning, conceptualizing, etc.).

HOW TO ENCOURAGE CHILDREN TO SOLVE PROBLEMS

Provide materials and allow time appropriate to the child's age and level of development in the areas of science, concepts of size, shape, texture, weight, color, etc., dramatic play, art, music, numerical concepts, spatial, locational and other relationships.

HOW TO PROMOTE LANGUAGE UNDERSTANDING

Some examples are:

1. Give children ample time to talk to each other and ask questions in the language of their choice.

2. Encourage free discussion and conversation between children and adults.

3. Provide games, songs, stories and poems which offer new and interesting vocabulary.

4. Encourage children to tell and listen to stories.

HOW TO WORK TOWARD RECOGNITION OF THE SYMBOLS FOR LETTERS AND NUMBERS

Make use of information that is relevant to the child's interests, such as his name, telephone number, address and age. Make ample use of written language within the context of the child's understanding. For example, experience personal stories, make name labels and discuss signs that are familiar.

HOW TO ENCOURAGE CHILDREN TO ORGANIZE THEIR EXPERIENCES AND UNDERSTAND CONCEPTS

The sequence of classroom activities should progress from simple to more complex tasks, and from concrete to abstract concepts. Activities can be organized around concepts to be learned.

HOW TO PROVIDE A BALANCED PROGRAM

Although each day's activities should be planned by the staff, the schedule should allow ample time for both spontaneous activity by children and blocks of time for teacher-directed activities.

HOW TO PROMOTE PHYSICAL GROWTH

This can be accomplished through regular periods for physical activity (both indoor and out).

HOW TO PROVIDE APPROPRIATE GUIDANCE WHILE CHILDREN ARE USING EQUIPMENT AND MATERIALS

Staff should be actively involved with children during periods of physical activity. During such activities, staff should take opportunities to increase their contact with individual children. To ensure safety, activities should be adequately supervised.

HOW TO HAVE A CURRICULUM WHICH IS RELEVANT

This can be accomplished by including in each classroom materials and activities which reflect the cultural background of the children. Examples of materials include: books, records, posters, maps, charts, dolls, clothing. Activities may include celebration of cultural events and holidays, serving foods related to other cultures, stories, music and games representative of children's background, and inviting persons who speak the child's native language to assist with activities.

HOW TO INCLUDE PARENTS

Parents can be valuable resources in planning activities which reflect the children's heritage. Teachers may request suggestions from parents on ways to integrate cultural activities into the program. For example, parents may wish to: plan holiday celebrations, prepare foods unique to various cultures, recommend books, records or other materials for the classroom, act as classroom volunteers, suggest games, songs and art projects which reflect cultural customs.

HOW TO PROVIDE HEALTH EDUCATION FOR CHILDREN

Activities to integrate educational aspects of other components into the daily education program could include: time to talk about physical and dental examinations in order to increase understanding and reduce fears, books and pictures about doctors and dentists, materials for dramatic play (stethoscope, nurse's uniform, flashlight), role playing before and after visits to doctors, dentists, hospitals, clinics, etc., assistance in meal preparation, setting table, learning experiences though food preparation (adding liquids to solids, seasoning, freezing, melting, heating, cooling, cooking simple foods), books, pictures, films, trips related to the source of foods (farm, garden, warehouse, market, grocery store).

HOW TO PROVIDE ENHANCED UNDERSTANDING BETWEEN PARENTS AND STAFF

The plan should indicate some of the ways parents and staff will work together to understand each child and provide for his learning experiences. The plan should include details of ways the home and center will attempt to supplement each other in providing positive experiences for the child. Procedures should be established to facilitate maximum communication between staff and parents. Examples: newsletters, parent/teacher conferences, group meetings, phone calls, home visits, posters, bulletin boards, radio/TV announcements, orientation and training sessions, designing activities for children at home. Have the parent participate in classroom/center activities. Also provide parents with workshops, publications and special referrals, etc.

(This section is reprinted with permission (1987) from Head Start Performance Standards, Department of Health and Human Services, Publication OHD 84-31131.)

TOOLBOX TIPS

"When a family selects a child care center, they are not simply buying a service that allows them to work. They are buying an environment that determines in large part the development of their children."

Psychology Today
Credit: Edward F. Zigler,
Yale University

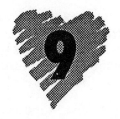

CHILD SAFETY

SAFETY FIRST

Rules and regulations vary from state to state. This is just an example of some rules. Check with the licensing bureau before proceeding.

1. Indoor and outdoor space should be sufficient and appropriate for necessary program activities and for support functions (offices, food preparation, custodial services if they are conducted on the premises). In addition, rest/nap facilities and space for isolation of sick children should be available.

2. Radiators, stoves, hot water pipes, portable heating units and similar potential hazards are adequately screened or insulated to prevent burns.

3. No highly flammable furnishings or decorations shall be used.

4. Flammable and other dangerous materials and potential poisons shall be stored in locked cabinets or storage facilities accessible only to authorized persons. Cleaning supplies and potentially dangerous materials should be stored separately from food and out of reach of children.

5. Emergency lighting shall be available in case of power failure. High powered flashlights may be used. Candles are fire hazards.

6. Approved, working fire extinguishers shall be readily available. Adults in the program should be able to locate and properly operate fire extinguishers.

7. Indoor and outdoor premises shall be kept clean and free, on a daily basis, of undesirable and hazardous material and conditions. If evidence of rodents or vermin is found, the local health or sanitation departments may provide assistance or referral for exterminators. At regular intervals, programs should be checked for and corrected of splintered surfaces, extremely sharp or protruding corners or edges, loose or broken parts. All clear

glass doors should be clearly marked with opaque tape to avoid accidents.

8. Outdoor play areas shall be made so as to prevent children from leaving the premises and getting into unsafe and unsupervised areas. Where outdoor space borders on unsafe areas (traffic, streets, ponds, swimming areas) adults should always be positioned to supervise the children. If possible, such areas should be enclosed.

9. Paint coatings on premises used for care of children shall be determined to assure the absence of a hazardous quantity of lead. Old buildings may be dangerous. Be sure to check for lead contamination. The local public health department can be contacted to provide information on lead poisoning and to detect hazardous quantities of lead in the facility.

10. Rooms shall be well lighted. Fixtures which have a low glare surface to sufficiently diffuse and reflect light may be useful. Use bulbs with sufficient wattage. Check and replace burned-out bulbs regularly.

11. A source of water approved by the appropriate local authority shall be available in the facility. Adequate toilets and handwashing facilities shall be available and easily reached by children. Verify state and local licensing requirements in these areas.

12. All sewage and liquid waste shall be disposed of through a sewer system approved by an appropriate responsible authority, and garbage and trash shall be stored in a safe and sanitary manner until collected. Disposal problems can be referred to the local sanitation and public works department. Keep all waste materials away from children's activity areas and from areas used for storage and for preparation of food.

13. In many states, there shall be at least 35 square feet of indoor space per child available for the care of children (i.e., exclusive of bathrooms, halls, kitchen and storage places). There shall be at least 75 square feet per child outdoors. (This space regulation varies from state to state. Check with your own regulatory agency.) Where minimum space is not available, various alternatives can be considered. For example, a variation in program design could be to stagger the program day, the program week and outdoor play periods. In this manner, all children will not be present at the same time. In some cases, outdoor space requirements may be met by arranging for daily use of an adjoining or nearby school yard, park, playground, vacant lot or other space. Be sure that these areas are easily accessible and fulfill the necessary safety requirements. In some cases, it may be necessary to locate more suitable facilities. (Remember, check your own state regulations for specific square footage, playground regulations, etc.)

14. Adequate provisions shall be made for handicapped children to ensure their safety and comfort. Ramps, railings and special materials and equipment may be needed in order to allow such children maximum possible mobility. Community resources may be used to acquire needed special materials and services. Confirm compliance with all state and local licensing requirements.

(This section is reprinted with permission (1987) from Head Start Performance Standards, Department of Health and Human Services, Publication OHD 84-31131.)

KEEPING STAFF & KIDS HAPPY

TIPS ABOUT ORGANIZING DAY CARE PROGRAMS

Opening a day care center takes months of careful planning and organizing. Even if you are confident that you've thought of everything, one thing is certain: you haven't! Dozens of tiny problems will pop up to plague you in those first weeks and months of operation.

Here are some helpful hints that will help you to anticipate possible problem areas, and keep your center running smoothly.

STAFFING SUGGESTIONS

1. Take advantage of any training programs that are offered. One day care provider utilized her CPR and First Aid training to save a child's life.

2. Delegate chores to others and expect them to carry out their responsibilities. Assign jobs for lunch room duty, playground supervision, opening and closing the center, purchasing snacks, etc. Be sure to review job responsibilities with prospective employees so that they know all the tasks that are part of the job, even those that may be on a rotating basis.

3. Set priorities and recognize that everything will not be perfect.

4. When conflicts arise, you do not have to raise your voice. If you remain calm, the other people involved will respond to your calm command of the situation.

5. Employees in the center need a secure place to keep their personal belongings such as handbags and wallets. If desk drawers do not lock, make sure there is a closet available in the office or kitchen.

6. Don't stop at classified ads to recruit qualified workers. Reach out to all local social service agencies, attend job fairs, hand out job descriptions at child care conferences.

7. You may want to post job openings outside your facility, "Education Career Opportunities Available."

8. Good staff interview questions: What do you find challenging or stimulating about children? What kind and how much responsibility are you comfortable in assuming? What do you like about young children? What would you most like to learn to do that you can't do now? How would you discipline a three year old differently than a five year old? How would you handle a child who is tattling, biting, or destroying another child's art project? Discuss personnel policies regarding compensation, benefits, grievance procedures and probationary employment period. Your program philosophy should be clearly explained.

9. One of the most difficult problems for any day care administrator is finding qualified substitutes when regular staff members are absent. Consider forming a substitute pool with several other centers in your area. Each center shares in the cost to place classified ads; centers take turn screening applicants and updating lists. Because of the high turnover rate, lists must be updated at least once a month.

10. There are certain times of the day that are stressful. As you network with other center directors, you will discover their stress times and how they handle them. From experience, arrival and departure of children, naptime and mealtime seem to be more stressful. Hiring an extra person to help at these times may be desirable.

11. Take a few breaks during the day. While the children are napping or watching "Sesame Street," relax, so you have the stamina to face the challenges ahead.

12. Exercise helps the mind and body. Play music and twist and turn with the kids to relax.

13. Play dough is fun for adults too. It is therapeutic to pound and mold things along with the kids.

14. Learn to distinguish between essential and non-essential rules. Don't waste time and energy trying to enforce rules that really don't matter. (Example: Trying to make three year olds stand in straight lines. Who really cares?)

15. Visit a potential field trip location in advance of taking the children there to familiarize yourself with parking availability, picnic facilities, snack bar prices, bathroom locations and directions.

16. Plan field trips when it is not peak time for traffic. Children become restless when confined for an extended period of time.

SAFETY CONCERNS

17. Childproof your center. Remove items that are easily broken or dangerous if swallowed.

18. Crawl on the floor and you will see things that are hazardous to children from a child's perspective.

19. Be sure all employees and you know the location of the fire extinguisher and how to operate it. Plan a fire escape route and practice a fire drill several times a year.

20. Remove barrettes from a little girl's hair during naptime if you think they could be removed by the child and put into her mouth.

21. Tell parents about any medical situation or injury no matter how slight. A bloody nose, vomiting, accident, temperature or a bee sting will sound 100% more serious if the child tells the parents before you do.

22. Balloons are not recommended. Broken pieces could be swallowed.

23. Using a portable telephone if you must take a call will allow you to continue to supervise the children.

24. Keep changing supplies above the changing table where they will be out of the children's reach. Many ointments and creams are toxic if swallowed, and the outer plastic liner of disposable diapers can also be hazardous if placed over the head.

25. In case of accidents, keep a bag of kitty litter to absorb liquids and mask odors (easily vacuumed or swept up, too).

PLAY AREAS - INDOORS AND OUTDOORS

26. Rooms can be color coded and decorated to signal functionally different space uses. This will help children recognize the use and behavior appropriate for each area (quiet rooms, blue; play areas, yellow; etc.).

27. To prevent trips and bumps, locate your block area away from traffic flow and never by a door. Have adequate shelf space to store all blocks.

28. A good way to organize block storage is to trace each type of block, cut out the shapes and tape them to the edge of the storage shelf. At clean-up time, children just match the shapes to put the blocks away neatly.

29. When planning gardens and new landscaping around the center, choose a variety of trees and shrubs that change with the seasons. Children will be able to observe first hand the passage of time by watching dogwoods flower in spring, become lush green in summer, and blazing red in autumn. (Caution: make sure none of the plants are poisonous.) The State Cooperative Extension Service or local nursery/garden centers can help you design your plantings.

30. Make sure outside play area has water source to wash hands, clean tricycles and provide water for drinking and projects. Consider drainage facilities and/or basins to catch used water to avoid mud problems. Putting medium-sized stone under faucets will help prevent water pooling and mud.

31. Purchase high quality wooden toys and institutional bikes, tricycles and wagons. Although they are appreciably more expensive than the plastic models available in toy stores, they will last five times as long and

save you money in the long run. The Little Tikes play equipment is my recommendation for the outdoor playground. Their equipment includes durable slides, climbing apparatus, playhouses, etc. They are, in my opinion, safer than the swings and slides found at most elementary schools. Safety is jeopardized in many centers when children accidentally move in front of swings, slide exits, etc. You can prevent many accidents and collisions by purchasing low to the ground activity equipment such as Little Tikes. (A free early childhood Playground Planning Kit is offered by Environments, Inc. 800-EI-CHILD.)

32. The U.S. Consumer Product Safety Commission offers a free booklet, titled *A HANDBOOK FOR PUBLIC PLAYGROUND SAFETY*. To obtain a copy, send a postcard request to: U.S. Consumer Product Safety Commission, Midwestern Regional Office, 230 South Dearborn Street, Room 2944, Chicago, IL 60604 (312-353-8260).

FOOD AND HEALTH TIPS

33. Contact the state licensing bureau or the Child Care Food Program for nutritious meal planning ideas and suggestions for snacks.

34. The licensing bureau is also a good source for information on food programs and training, or for supplies.

35. Plan meals and snacks and purchase needed items in advance. Leaving the center to obtain forgotten items is a waste of time and energy, as well as a risk if the center is short-staffed.

36. Keeping your center healthy is advantageous to all. To reduce the spread of germs, air the rooms daily, use disposable diapers and wash your hands after changing babies and before serving meals. Disinfect the changing area, toys and play equipment with a sanitizing solution such as LYSOL® cleaner and spray at the end of each day to reduce the spread of germs. When parents visit your center, they are very aware of the smell. Day care personnel often "get used to" diaper smell. By keeping the air fresh, and the center clean and germ-free, your center will present the best impression.

37. Disposable gloves and disposable diapers are recommended to use when changing babies. See a report published by the American Academy of Pediatrics, titled *1991 Red Book: Report of the Committee on Infectious Diseases*. This report details diapering procedures that minimize contamination of children, caregivers and environmental surfaces and objects in a child care program. Also see *Caring for Our Children: National Health and Safety Performance Standards for Out-of-Home Child Care Programs*. Diapering standards are discussed by the experts of the American Academy of Pediatrics and the American Public Health Association. Refer to the Appendix for information on obtaining these publications.

38. Wash hands in a bathroom sink after diapering a baby, not in the sink where food preparation is involved. Disposable diapers involve less handling and leakage. They are recommended by the American Academy of Pediatrics for use in day care centers.

39. Establish routine cleaning schedules for all areas including classrooms, kitchen, office, bathrooms and storage areas. Decide which

tasks need to be done daily (sweeping, wiping tables); weekly (sanitizing infant toys with LYSOL® or a similar disinfectant); and monthly (cleaning kitchen cabinets and office shelves). Post appropriate lists in each area.

40. Keep a spray bottle filled with bleach solution (1/4 cup in 1 gallon of water) or LYSOL® in a storage area above the changing table. A quick spray after each change will sanitize the area and help eliminate germs. Diaper rash can be lessened by using disposable diapers and changing frequently so that the moisture does not irritate the baby's skin. (Store all cleaning supplies in a locked cabinet not accessible to the children.)

DAY-TO-DAY OPERATIONS

41. Children are individuals and should not have a rigidly structured day. Follow a schedule that is flexible. This is different from following a routine, which all of us need to some degree (see Hint 42).

42. Follow a daily routine so the children know what to expect. For example, "After we wake up from our nap, we have a snack and then we play and then my mom comes for me."

43. Don't offer ordinary day care. Give special attention to each child. Find a few minutes each day to interact one-on-one with each boy and girl. Hold them, hug them. Tell them how much their mom and dad love them and also how glad you are that they come to your center.

44. Avoid telling the kids to "hurry up." They are only little kids who are dealing with a different lifestyle than what we knew as children.

45. Talk about feelings when they appear disappointed, sad, hurt or just out of sorts. Children can be depressed too. A sick pet or relative causes anxiety. You may want to share this interaction with the child's parents.

46. Remember what it is like to be a child. Loud noises, harsh voices and a temperamental and impatient adult are unpleasant situations for children.

PARENTS AND POLICIES

47. Be clear when discussing policies on payments, sickness, vacation schedules and hours of operation with the parents. Put these items in writing and give each parent a copy.

48. The parents are interviewing you but it is important for you to interview them. You do not want every child in your program. Your intuition may tell you that your philosophy on children would be at odds with a particular parent. Be honest, professional, selective but not discriminatory. Let parents know that you will inform them of any difficulties their child may be experiencing.

49. Many providers build a trial period of two weeks into their initial agreement. This is for both you and the child/parent.

50. Keep a daily chart that shares information on the child's eating and napping habits. Parents want to know the day's happenings—what their child ate, drank, felt like, how she napped, diaper changes, general mood, etc.

51. Establish a parents' corner with a bulletin board to advertise upcoming events or to list the day's happenings. Remember a two year old can't always tell mommy what he did today. This is also a great place for a small lending library of books and pamphlets related to parenting. Be sure parents sign out library materials.

52. When you give a parent a tour of your center, show the indoor space, rest rooms for children, kitchen, lunch room, resource room, playground area, napping room, etc. Be completely open so they feel they really know all about the center.

53. Invite the parents to join the group for some activities. Parents can occasionally take an hour or two off to make cookies or go to the park.

54. Tell the parents that you welcome toys and baby equipment when they no longer need them and if they are still in very good condition.

55. Ask parents to contribute ideas for the center newsletter. Choose one topic each month (for example: bedtime battles, kindergarten readiness, bathroom training or super snacks) and ask parents for their favorite hints.

56. Ideally, there should be a place for parents to sit and wait for their child at pick-up time.

BUSINESS SENSE

57. Child care is challenging and you earn every penny that you are paid. Don't set your fee too low or it will be difficult to increase later on.

58. Research what the competition is charging to provide child care. In many areas, day care centers charge more than day care homes. A variety of rates are charged depending on the services and programs provided: infant care, toddler care, preschool, part-time care, kindergarten, before/after school, drop-in baby-sitting, summer camp for school age, handicapped or special needs children, intergenerational, sick care, etc. Compare prices for the services you will offer.

59. Decide ahead of time how many weeks you will allow a parent to miss tuition payments, and stick to it! A parent who can't pay $70 or $80 is even less likely to be able to pay $200. When I first opened my center, I allowed several parents (in the midst of unexpected economic crises) to build up hefty bills because I felt sorry for the children involved. Unfortunately, all my altruism earned me was several $1,000's in uncollectible debts. I learned my lesson the hard way.

60. You may give a price break when there are two children enrolled from one family. Only give a slight reduction in payment.

61. It may be tempting to enroll an extra child or two but you will probably regret it. Don't admit more children than you are legally permitted. Politely but firmly refuse to take on more children even if it is for a good friend or relative.

62. Imagine placing your own child in your center. Would you leave your child in a setting like this?

63. Network with day care providers. Exchange tips for managing time, space, children and parents. Talking about work with other people involved in the same profession keeps your spirits up. I recommend that you order my book *Start Your Own At-Home Child Care Business,* published by Doubleday. Although the title says "at-home," the ideas presented work well with both home and center day care with no overlap of information. The book is a companion to this one. Both books present valuable information and different ideas. Call 215-364-1945 for more information or to place an order (Visa and MasterCard accepted).

64. Post photos of all staff members; include their names, class assignments, and the hours they are in the center.

65. Never leave yourself open for charges of abuse. Document all accidents, even those considered minor. Record date, time, place, all adults present, witnesses and appropriate action taken.

66. Keep a list of names and numbers of all those who made telephone inquiries for child care and follow them up, if necessary. (Are you still interested? Did you find alternate care? If so, what made that other center more attractive?)

67. Call local newspapers and find out the name of the city editor or reporter on your beat. Then make sure that person gets a news release or black and white captioned photo at least once a month of your center's activities or involvement in community projects. (Order *Start Your Own At-Home Child Care Center* by Patricia Gallagher for more marketing ideas ($15.50). Call 215-364-1945, Visa and MasterCard accepted.)

68. When planning brochures, omit information that is likely to fluctuate often (fee schedules, faculty names). This information can be included in a photocopied insert so the brochures will not become obsolete as fast.

69. Good places to distribute pamphlets and registration information are real estate and relocation services offices, children's clothing stores, public libraries, employment agencies and churches/synagogues.

70. When ordering supplies through catalogs, always calculate the shipping costs. Many times the supplies you thought were a bargain may actually cost more than those from a higher priced manufacturer who ships merchandise free.

71. Find out if any local school districts are planning to hold surplus furniture and equipment auctions. This is a great way to pick up extra tables, chairs or audio-visual equipment. I once purchased a near perfect copier for $25. A friend of mine got an entire 300 piece set of wooden blocks for $50.

72. Good fundraising ideas: sponsor a children's flea market or used kid's clothing sale. Bake sales and children's activity days are also easy to organize and help generate income. They provide good public relations also.

73. Make sure your fundraising is cost-effective. If it takes fifty hours and twenty parents to organize a book sale and the center only nets $100, it might just be easier to raise tuition $1 a week.

74. You will receive better fundraising support if you try to raise money for a specific goal (new playground equipment, a field trip fund). Money raised by parents should directly benefit their children.

75. For information on modular day care centers contact Scotsman Buildings Modular Structures (800-472-2020). They offer a modular day care center delivered to your location. I have seen the buildings constructed by this company and they are beautifully designed and immediately functional.

76. Clarify the grouping category as defined by your licensing bureau. In many states, the age groups are:

infant:	birth through 12 months
young toddler:	13 through 24 months
older toddler:	25 through 36 months
preschool child:	37 months through the date the child enters first grade
young school-age child:	first grade through third grade
older school-age child:	fourth grade through fifteen years of age
volunteer:	a person sixteen years of age or older who is not included in the regulatory ratio and who assists in activities under the supervision of a staff person.

100 WAYS TO KEEP KIDS HAPPY

A child needs a warm, loving relationship with an adult that shows unconditional love. Make sure that you make the time to offer affection and encouragement. It is mutually rewarding to read, play games and even watch television with children. Some ideas that will create happy memories and also provide activities that contribute to the emotional and intellectual growth of children from infants through elementary age follow. Tips 1-49 apply primarily to infants, toddlers and preschoolers. Tips 50-100 are more appropriate for school-age children. But remember that children develop at their own pace, and many activities can be easily adapted for other age groups.

PRESCHOOL IDEAS

1. Take time to answer their endless questions.

2. Act silly with them sometimes. Show them your sense of spirit & fun.

3. Praise frequently.

4. Start a scrapbook of "Fun Times."

5. Make paper decorations using construction paper and odds and ends. Decorate for a special day called "Red Day." Serve a red snack, tell a story about *Little Red Riding Hood*, hide items that are red that the children have to look for, etc.

6. Make chains from paper.

7. Have an "un-birthday party" complete with a fancy cake, party treats and ice cream sundaes to celebrate everybody's "un-birthday."

8. Hang crepe paper streamers vertically from the top of a door to create a stage effect. Children love to peek through to sing songs or act out a play.

9. Pretend to fly an airplane over the neighborhood. What do you see from this vantage point?

10. Make a collage with colored cupcake papers.

11. On a snowy day, make angels in the fresh snow. Lay on your back in the snow and move your arms up and down (towards your head and feet) to make an angel impression.

12. Act out favorite nursery rhymes or fairy tales.

13. Change the endings of well known stories. Vary the story by using the child's name instead of Goldilock's. Change it to Katelyn and The Three Bears and use the child's name throughout the storytelling.

14. Make a train with chairs lined in a row. Tear up pieces of paper for tickets.

15. Give the children various household items and let them separate them into baskets or shopping bags filled with "big things" and "little things," or "kitchen things" and "bathroom things," etc.

16. Fill a plastic squeeze bottle with water and squirt the driveway, water the grass, or enjoy a cold drink!

17. Take a cassette player with story and song tapes along on trips in the car.

18. Wet the children's feet in a bucket of water. Make a trail of footprints on the pavement. Children hop or skip along delighting in the wet trail of footprints that they have created.

19. Cash register receipts are great for playing "store" or for lining up end to end to make a trail that the children follow.

20. Make a masking tape "balance beam" outside by putting tape on the sidewalk. Ask the children to walk steadily along the tape without falling off.

21. Draw a hopscotch game on the pavement using colored chalk.

22. Draw a hopscotch game on the back of an old vinyl tablecloth for an indoor game of hopscotch. Place on the floor and let the children enjoy hopping from one number to the next.

23. Candy sprinkles in a shaker bottle are great to decorate a store-bought cupcake.

24. Collect droppers from empty bottles. Show the children how it works and let them practice by transferring water from one container into another.

25. Freeze Kool-Aid®, JELL-O® and other juices in ice cube trays and other shaped containers for interesting treats.

26. Add food coloring to a glass of cold milk. You can make special days and holidays even more special by using this hint. For example, make green milk for Saint Patrick's Day and red for Valentine's Day.

27. Collect a variety of "rare rocks" as you walk around the playground or backyard. You can even decorate them for paperweight gifts for holidays or make "pet rocks."

28. Decorate small lunch bags to make your own "party bags."

29. Buy a box of a hundred or so paper cups and have the children line them up side by side, on top of each other, and upside down. Use wooden, spring-type clothespins to connect one to the other.

30. Save containers from 35mm film. Spread the containers on the floor. Have the children form shapes by placing the containers in a circle, triangle, rectangle or square.

31. Introduce a new letter such as R and sample foods that begin with R such as rice, raspberries, ring bologna and radishes.

32. Buy pre-baked cookies and ice with canned frosting. Add a few chocolate bits for eyes, nose and mouth and a little coconut for hair.

33. Take a walk and touch the tree branches, feel the bark, smell the flowers, examine the veins on the leaves.

34. Clap your hands if I say something silly such as "a cow barks" or "a duck growls."

35. Make a train by tying scarves together and "pulling" the children for a ride.

36. Try to carry a variety of objects on a large serving spoon. Then carry things on a small spoon. Also point out the difference between heavy and light such as a cotton ball versus an egg (hardboiled, of course).

37. On a piece of cardboard, draw a large capital letter. Dribble some Elmer's glue on the letter. Allow to dry and harden. The children can learn letters by tracing over the hardened letter surface.

38. Ask children for ideas for meals and snacks. Then, as a group, plan, cook, serve and clean up their feast.

39. Give children three or four toys or household items. Act out a story using those items.

40. Show the letters printed on a cereal box or can in your cupboard. Have children try to copy the letters.

41. Use scraps of wallpaper squares from a wallpaper book to make stepping stones. Children leap from one stone to the other trying not to fall in the water (the space between the wallpaper squares).

42. Use permanent ink markers to make a road or race track on an old

vinyl shower curtain or vinyl tablecloth. Use matchbox cars and narrate a tour of the neighborhood.

43. Name all of the things in which you can ride.

44. Tape record the children's conversation. Play it back for them.

45. Mix oil, water and food coloring in a clear bottle. Observe what happens.

46. Look out the window. Name all of the things that you see or all of the things that begin with a certain letter, or that grow, or fly, etc.

47. Put old blankets and sheets over a table and some chairs and make a fort.

48. Make an obstacle course by having the children go around a chair, crawl under a table, knock three times on a door, jump over a throw rug, etc.

49. Use old greeting cards to make bookmarks, collages or new original cards that you send to someone special.

SCHOOL AGE IDEAS

50. Nutshell Racers-Make tiny animals out of halved walnut shells. Paint or glue on apple ears, tails, etc. Insert a marble under the shell (do not glue) and race down a slanted board.

51. Both boys and girls of this age love to make and wear jewelry. Glue tiny alphabet macaroni on popsicle sticks or cardboard shapes to make name pins or tags for bookbags, etc. Roll tiny beads from salt dough (1 cup flour, 1/2 cup salt, water to moisten); use a toothpick to make a tiny hole through each bead. After beads harden, paint with enamel paints or nail polish and string to make necklaces and bracelets.

52. Encourage free reading by establishing an after-school or summer book club. Designate a specific quiet time each day when everyone (including teachers and aides) reads or looks at magazines.

53. Organize a surprise book swap. Each child brings in a good used book from home wrapped in a brown paper bag. Books are placed in a large box and each child gets to choose a new book. (Teacher should be prepared with a few extras for those children who invariably forget their books.)

54. Prepare a "Time Capsule" of things the children feel represent their world today. Include pictures, old toys, stories and newspaper clippings. Place the material in a large glass jar and bury it on your property. Draw a map to the site and decide where to store it (the map) so that people in future years (10? 25?) will find the map and locate the "Time Capsule."

55. Play balloon volleyball. Stretch a string across the room, use a balloon instead of a ball, and players must stay on their knees! (Balloons should only be used with older children.)

56. If you have access to a video camera, let children make their own music videos. First they must choose the song, then design a backdrop and

costumes and practice lip-syncing. Finally, record the video and plan a "dance" party so everyone gets to view the videos.

57. Have fun brainstorming. It gets the children used to thinking quickly and creatively and helps with their problem solving abilities. When brainstorming, select a specific question or problem and set a reasonable time limit. Remember, there are no wrong or silly answers when you brainstorm—every response is acceptable. Afterward you may wish to go back and decide which responses (critical thinking) are "do-able" and which are impossible or impractical. Sample brainstorming questions: a. things to do with a rubber band; b. the scariest things in the world; c. things that could be used for Halloween makeup; d. ways to keep your little brother or sister out of your toys; e. good presents for your parents.

58. If you have an out-of-the-way corner, keep a large jigsaw puzzle under construction there at all times. Some children will wander over, place a piece and then leave. Others will concentrate for long periods of time. Great fun for all to see the picture emerge. (Two large aluminum cookie sheets cut and taped together make a good puzzle tray. Try to find the kind with sides so that puzzle pieces don't go wandering.)

59. NEVER appoint team captains and allow them to choose sides for a game or activity. YOU already know who will be chosen last, so please spare those children the heartache by picking teams by colors, numbers, etc.

60. Plan a field trip to a familiar and close place (the kitchen, bathroom, playground, supply closet). Have one child act as tour guide and point out all the interesting features. Try to concentrate on things you've never noticed before.

61. Keep a picture file that children may refer to when they are drawing or writing stories. (How do I draw a cat? What can I say about the mountains?)

62. Teach kids to sew. A scrap bag of material and buttons, along with a supply of needles and thread, provides hours of fun.

63. Collect a "million" (bottle caps, sea shells, paper clips). As children add to the collection, keep a running total. Kids will be amazed at how much a million actually is.

64. Make a family or class cookbook. Have children contribute their favorite recipes, maybe even draw step-by-step instructions.

65. Once a week, instead of snacktime, have "tea time." Serve hot or iced tea (herb tea if you are worried about caffeine) and fancy sandwiches or cookies. Put on some classical music or read aloud from a classic story (*Oliver Twist, The Wind in the Willows*).

66. Introduce children to the Broadway stage. Have a featured musical of the week. Tell the story, then listen to the album (a few songs each day).

67. Change rules to familiar games to make them more interesting, challenging or just sillier. Play kickball, but run the bases backward; play dodgeball with a big, wet sponge; play indoor basketball with buckets and rolled-up socks.

68. Kids love scavenger hunts. Make up lists of items to find at home or in school, inside and out. The team which collects the most items on their list, wins.

69. Let the kids be in charge! Give each child a chance to teach a new game or craft to the group. You can help by providing idea books or children's magazines for them to look through.

70. Mix up your meals. Have pizza for breakfast and cereal for lunch. Talk about why we think certain foods can only be eaten at a certain time of day.

71. Each week, invite someone to your center as the "Secret Storyteller." This can be a parent, friend, neighbor or one of the children. Change the time each week, so the children will never know when the storyteller is coming, and let the guest choose a favorite book or story to share with the group.

72. When it snows, let children "paint" the snow with colored water in spray bottles or old detergent bottles.

73. Use the Sunday comics as bright, inexpensive wrapping paper for children's gifts.

74. Never punish a child by making him or her WRITE. Writing should be a joyous activity—a means of self-expression and a way to work out feelings and problems. It should not be associated with drudgery and boredom.

75. Make a cake from "scratch" and one from a mix. Compare taste, texture, ingredients and ease of preparation.

76. Conduct your own consumer taste tests. Which flavored drink mix do your kids really like best?

77. Plant an herb garden (herbs grow well indoors in pots, too) and dry herbs to give as holiday gifts.

78. Make face paints from powdered poster paint and cold cream. Apply with cotton swabs, just tissue off.

79. Make cookie houses out of graham crackers using frosting or icing as the "glue" to keep it together. Decorate with tiny candies, raisins, and pieces of dried fruit. Then eat!

80. Allow children solitude and privacy when they need it, but be aware of their actions.

81. Encourage children to examine the world from different points of view. How does a puddle look to a butterfly? A mouse? A dog? A boy on a bicycle? Write a story or draw a picture to illustrate your ideas.

82. Take a well-known song (like *Yankee Doodle*) and change the words. How many different versions can you make up?

83. Draw your own comic strip. Make up a super hero and give him or her special powers.

84. Soak minute-type rice in water tinted with food coloring. After rice is dry, use it to make collages on paper or wood. Cover a section with glue, pour on colored rice, and dump off the extra.

85. Keep a log of how many different birds (license plates, animals) you see in one week.

86. Visit the food store and pick out a food you've never tried before. Find out where it comes from and share a sample with the group.

87. Invite a different parent to come to the center each week and tell about his or her job or hobby.

88. Kids love to write stories on the typewriter. Garage sales are great places to pick up an inexpensive old portable.

89. Have a photo day, when everyone can bring in a camera and take pictures of their friends. They can also bring in silly props or clothing to make their pictures more imaginative.

90. Have everyone bring in a baby picture to display on the bulletin board. Don't tell who is who; let everyone guess.

91. Make a list of all the things in your house that your parents never heard of when they were young. (Microwave ovens, VCRs, video games.)

92. Make a bubble gum sculpture by chewing a big wad of gum, sticking it on a piece of cardboard and shaping it with toothpicks. (Don't chew it after you've played with it!)

93. Hold a pet show for stuffed animals. Give prizes for the biggest, littlest, funniest, dirtiest, oldest, etc.

94. Collect old buttons and make a collage.

95. Set up an obstacle course for your bicycles. Use chalk or masking tape to mark off the path. Paint empty gallon milk bottles (plastic) and orange juice containers and use as traffic cones.

96. Empty liter soda bottles make great bowling pins. Add a little sand to the bottles to make them more stable, and use a soft ball or medium-sized playground ball as a bowling ball.

97. Plan a Silly Olympics Day so that all children, even the non-athletic ones, will have a chance at winning. Make up events like raisin tossing, leapfrog relays, and tricycle races.

98. Plan a meal around a single food or idea (example: everything round: hamburgers, carrot slices, cookies; everything containing apples: chicken salad with apples, apple sauce and apple pie).

99. Teach children to estimate by holding a weekly contest to guess the number of beans in a jar, shells in a box, etc.

100. Buy a large bag of already popped popcorn and let the children build interesting structures by using toothpicks to connect one piece to another.

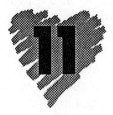

The Learning Environment

PLANNING A LEARNING ENVIRONMENT FOR INFANTS TO FIVES

L ucky for us, the days of having to improvise everything are over. New and unique materials exist that have been developed specifically for the early childhood field to meet the developmental needs of young children in group situations.

Durable, well-designed equipment is not inexpensive. This is truly an area where "you get what you pay for." Inexpensive equipment may sometimes end up costing you more because it will need frequent repair or replacement, or worse, can cause accidents. Things that are designed for home use often just don't hold up with the constant heavy use groups of children give them. Since dollars are never plentiful in this field, careful selection of equipment is very important.

HOW TO GET STARTED

If you are selecting equipment for a new center, you have a lot of decisions to make. You probably have a defined budget to stay within. There are certain "givens." You will need at least one child's chair for each preschooler in your center. You need at least that many places for children to sit at tables. You will need that many cots or rest mats as well if you are running a full-day program. Each child must also have cubby space, a place to hang his or her coat and put his personal belongings. But there are many variables. How many shelves for holding toys will you have? Will you have indoor as well as outdoor gross-motor equipment on which children can crawl and climb? What types of materials will you provide to add essential softness to your environment?

If you are adding equipment to an existing program you have different decisions to make. You need to decide what you have that is usable and then prioritize your needs. Survey what you already have. You could walk from room to room in your center and list things on paper. Or, if you have the energy, come in on a Saturday and have a work party (perhaps involving parents) to clean up, paint, fix up ... and throw out. Try pieces in different classrooms. Then list what is missing, things you would like that would enhance your program. Undoubtedly, you will have to pare down your "wish list." Make decisions about items based on their "play value" to children, flexibility, durability and attractiveness.

SAFETY

You have to think of the worst possible things that could happen to equipment, the worst possible misuse of it. Many safety hazards can be prevented by good adult supervision and intervention, but you have to think about what could happen if someone had his or her back turned. All equipment in child care centers should comply with Consumer Product Safety Guidelines. Wooden materials should not break or splinter easily. There should be no sharp or rough edges that could scratch children. Paint should be nontoxic. Large pieces should not tip over under ordinary or even extraordinary circumstances. (Children will climb on things that were not designed for climbing.) There should be no possibility for children to get their heads stuck. If there is plastic in the material, it should be the kind that is not brittle and would not break to form sharp edges or points. There should be no glass. Equipment that appears in reputable early childhood supply catalogs is usually prescreened for safety. These things are especially important to keep in mind when using home-made or improvised equipment.

DURABILITY

Check to see that furniture is sturdy and well-made. Do doors on play equipment hang straight and open and close smoothly? Joints should not be loose. Fabric or vinyl fabric should be well-cut with tight seams. It is in the durability area that many "variety-store toys" are unsatisfactory. Even though a riding toy or child's table may cost less, you will not save money because the toy is more likely to fall apart or break with heavy use.

CLEANABILITY

Equipment should be easy to clean for both aesthetics and hygiene. (Diapers leak and you will find you will often have to clean the surfaces of toys and equipment. Disposable diapers with elastic bands are best for children in day care centers.) Children get things dirty quickly, especially in good programs that allow children to dig in sand, paint and engage in other messy learning activities. It should be possible for you or other caregivers to clean surfaces with a damp sponge and the occasional use of a mild cleanser. (I always used a disinfectant such as LYSOL®.) Preventing the spread of germs is a serious responsibility of child care providers. It should be possible to clean surfaces frequently with disinfecting solutions without damaging them.

USABILITY WITH DIFFERENT AGES

If you can move equipment from one room to another in your program, you can give both children and staff a lift. There is nothing like a change of scenery. Also, in all practicality, children are often moved into a different room at the end of the day, often a room planned for a different age. Equipment that is safe for little ones as well as interesting and challenging for older ones will get a lot of use and your money will be well-spent.

MOVABILITY

Early childhood classrooms are not static places. Teachers and even children should be able to move equipment easily to rearrange their own rooms and create their own new spaces. If you can bring equipment outside easily, you will get added play value from the equipment.

DEVELOPMENTAL APPROPRIATENESS

The equipment should match the children who will be using it. If the children cannot reach the pedals on the tricycle, that tricycle is not developmentally appropriate. A balance beam is not appropriate for children who are not yet walking. Small riding toys and shape boxes are not appropriate for a bright group of five-year-olds ready to explore the world. It boils down to knowing what the emerging skills are for the age in question and the children can practice those skills.

TABLES AND CHAIRS

Tables and chairs should be the right height for the age group. Children should be able to sit on chairs with their feet on the floor and the table should be waist or mid-chest height. Tables with adjustable legs are the best bet for child-care centers. That gives you the flexibility to move a table to a different room and adjust it to the height appropriate for the children in that room.

You need table space for eating. But you also need table space for some interest-center play particularly art, science and fine-motor toys. A table in the library/language development corner might also be desirable, and you will need a place to put the record player and musical instruments (although a shelf could be used for this). Tables can, of course, be used for many purposes. Tables come in many shapes-square, rectangle, round, horseshoe, trapezoid. Combining different shapes of several smaller tables gives you greater flexibility in room arrangement than using large tables. Smaller tables also encourage small group activities and can be used more easily in interest centers.

Look for sturdy, "industrial-strength" tables that do not wobble. Formica tops or other smooth, easily cleanable surfaces are a must. If the bottoms of the legs have flexible knob ends, these can make up for small irregularities in floor surfaces. Also look for tables with rounded corners to minimize the damage from inevitable mishaps and falls.

Chairs, likewise, should be the right height for the children who will be using them. They come in all different sizes, even very short so that toddlers can sit with their feet on the floor. Children's coordination at table-toy tasks and while eating will be much better if their feet are anchored on solid ground. Don't forget about adult chairs. Adults deserve a degree of comfort, too, and sitting with your knees at your ears may not be the best way to achieve this! (Not that early childhood teachers have much opportunity to sit around!) Keep portability in mind with chairs, too. Children, especially two-year-olds, like to carry chairs around, make trains and generally rearrange things. The surfaces should be smooth for easy cleaning with a disinfectant such as LYSOL. Stackability of chairs is another thing to think about. Chairs should never be stacked in a room where children are playing, for safety reasons, but stackability can be handy for the cleaning people.

SHELVES

It's hard to have too many shelves. Early childhood teachers never seem to have enough. Every teacher will have her or his own ideas, but generally it is advisable to have at least seven or eight shelves per classroom: two for the block corner-one for blocks, one for vehicles and accessories; at least one for dramatic play to hold shoes, purses, boxes and props; one for art supplies; one or two for manipulatives and math toys; one for science materials; one for books; and one for language development toys.

Shelves should be low and open to allow easy access for children. Children should be able to reach their own toys and put them away again. Since children sometimes climb on shelves when the teacher isn't looking, it is essential that they are sturdy and secured so that they can not fall on a child.

INDOOR GROSS-MOTOR EQUIPMENT

People usually think of their outside playground as their "gross-motor area." However, there are few places in the country where the weather is so perfect that you can count on going outside every day. Also, children don't stop needing to use their large muscles simply because they are inside. They need to have safe pieces of equipment on which to crawl, climb, jump and slide indoors. (If you don't provide for this, children will climb on tables, chairs and shelves, often causing accidents.)

All children need a legitimate place to release energy. If you work with special-needs children, and more and more special-needs children are being integrated into regular preschool programs, indoor gross-motor equipment is especially important for building muscle tone and balance.

There are many excellent gross-motor pieces designed for early childhood environments. It is best to find pieces with multiple uses. Again, make the developmental match, find pieces that meet the skill level of children who will be using them.

CRAWLING

There are large, soft, vinyl-covered foam shapes for infants and toddlers to crawl and climb on that eliminate the possibility of injury if they lose their balance. Some have Velcro on them so they can be arranged and rearranged in many different ways, providing new challenges. (These pieces are greatly enjoyed by older children as well and add delightful elements of softness and color to the classroom.) One such example is on the front cover of this book!

Collapsible tunnels and modular pieces that fit together to form hollow cubes and tunnels also encourage children to crawl and move through spaces.

When children crawl and explore spaces they are learning a lot about their bodies-where they fit, what they can do, and they are also learning about the concepts of space and location.

CLIMBING

Climbing is an ongoing need of children from about eighteen months on. Wooden climbers come in different sizes and most are collapsible for storage. Check them for stability. Climbers for toddlers and twos should not be adjustable in height. Be sure to use cushioning mats under wooden climbers.

RIDING

Riding toys are appropriate indoors as well as outdoors. Toddlers and twos absolutely love small-wheeled toys that they propel with their feet on the ground. Teachers might section off one area of their rooms for riding toys. Try creating a track or road for these toys using tape on the floor.

If you have the space, especially if there is a "gross-motor room" in your center (very desirable), older children will enjoy using tricycles, wagons, and "haulers" indoors.

ROCKING

Children also love rocking boats. They provide "vestibular motion," as do rocking chairs and other toys that rock back and forth. They are also good pro-social toys, because they only work well when two or more children are using them. They encourage children to cooperate and have fun together and can help lead children from solitary play toward cooperative play.

ART AND SENSORY PLAY

You will need easels and drying racks for your art corner. Painting at the easel is a very valuable early childhood experience and should be offered to children daily. Children can be taught to be quite independent at the easel, but this activity still needs supervision. Easels come in several interesting designs and are all collapsible for easier storage. There are three-way easels, the traditional double easels, wall easels that take up minimal space, even clear Plexiglass easels. Most have chalkboard faces, giving them multiple uses. Paint trays should be removable to allow for easy cleaning.

Sand and water tables can facilitate play with these important materials. It is desirable to have one for each classroom. Some have a wooden top so they can double as a table. Others are made of clear plastic so children can see under the surface of the water from the outside of the table. Water tables should be easily movable and have drains so they are easy to empty.

DRAMATIC PLAY

The basics for encouraging extremely important dramatic play in an early childhood environment include your typical "housekeeping" furniture: stove, sink, refrigerator, table and chairs, and doll bed. Don't neglect to have the table and chairs because that is where a lot of the "action" takes place. Durability is very important. Look for hard-woods, heavy-duty hardware and magnetic catches on doors.

There are many exciting extras available in catalogs. One of the most interesting new things is modular soft furniture to create a "living room." They are large cushions of varying shapes and sizes covered with colorful vinyl-coated nylon. Children can take them apart and rearrange them to make couches, easy chairs, even beds. This piece of equipment has an added advantage: it encourages flexibility in children's thinking.

Puppet stages, "store fronts," playhouses, phone booths and other dramatic play catalysts are great additions if your budget and space allow.

BLOCKS

No early childhood setting is complete without blocks. There are many types of blocks available that help you match the developmental level of children.

Hardwood "unit blocks" are the most familiar kind of blocks, and certainly basic for children three and older. The more blocks you provide and the more shapes you include, the more creative the building will be. Although blocks are expensive, they last forever and have great learning and play value for children. Accessories such as plastic animals, small people and vehicles will add to the dramatic play value of blocks.

An alternative to wooden blocks are large foam rubber blocks covered with colorful vinyl-coated nylon fabric. The main thing two-year-olds like to do with blocks is to stack them up so they can have the fun of knocking them down (cause and effect). When these soft blocks fall nobody gets hurt ... and they are almost noiseless! Toddlers and twos, in their "autonomy" stage of development, like to feel powerful. These large but light blocks allow them to feel strong and make something big. Older children also love these blocks and make large things to get inside of.

Large, wooden hollow blocks are also available and a great addition to classrooms of four- and five-year-olds. These blocks are used for both constructive play and dramatic play. Children usually work together and plan in order to make something big that they can really use for their own dramatic play. There are also large, colorful plastic blocks that fit together.

COTS AND CUBBIES

Each child should have his own space in a cubby for clothing and personal belongings. This serves not only a housekeeping function, but also to make each child feel important and special. Use your own best judgement when it comes to the placement or formation of shelving, wall units, wall systems, cubbies, stacking arrangements and any structure in your center. All items must be bolted or secured in some fashion so that there is no possibility that children could become stuck or tip over equipment.

If you run a full-day program, you will need rest cots or mats. Check your state licensing requirements, because some states require that children be elevated off the floor on cots. The main disadvantage of cots is they are bulky when stored and can be unwieldy to move around. Vinyl-covered foam mats take up less space and are generally more comfortable. Each child must have his own labelled cot or mat for health reasons. Cots and mats should have easily cleanable surfaces that are not damaged by wiping with LYSOL or a similar type of disinfectant. Some mats fold for easy storage, others hang on a wall system.

PLANNING YOUR CLASSROOM ENVIRONMENT

In child care settings, where children and adults spend many hours together engaged in learning and play, it is important that the environment of the classroom be attractive and organized. The types of furniture, toys, and equipment you have, how they are arranged in the space of your room and what you do to remain organized influences the smooth functioning of your program.

The benefit of a well organized environment is that children work more independently, with less conflict and greater concentration. Instead of spending most of your time managing children's behavior or looking for materials, you will have more time to interact with one or two children at a time. Not only can a well planned environment facilitate a good learning program, it can be part of your learning program as well. Children can learn many skills from their environment.

1. Independence. A frequently stated goal of early childhood programs is to develop independence in children. Children should gradually learn to do things themselves, without assistance from an adult. Toys can be stored within easy reach so that children don't have to ask the adult for everything. There can be a designated space and container for toys so that they are easy to find and children will know where to put them back. A simple sign-up system can help children plan ahead, make choices and

know that their choices will be respected.

2. A sense of order. The "interest center" classroom organization groups toys of similar function or learning focus together. Even the youngest children can sense this order. Children will figure out that, in this room, books go in one place, dolls in another, and blocks somewhere else.

3. Aesthetics. When children are exposed to well-designed toys and equipment, beautiful wood, pleasing colors and exquisite illustrations, they learn to appreciate quality in playthings.

4. A sense of pride. When a teacher takes the time to make a classroom beautiful, especially when children are involved in the process, and children's work is displayed attractively, children become proud of the place in which they spend their time. This can be seen at open-house events, when children eagerly drag their parents into their own classrooms and point out things with pride.

SOME BASIC PRINCIPLES OF ROOM ARRANGEMENT

How you arrange your space will depend on several considerations: the placement of your carpeted area and hard flooring, where the windows are, where the doors are, where the water is located and the shape of the room. Here are some guidelines.

1. Separate quiet areas from noisy, active play areas. Blocks, dramatic play, woodworking and gross motor play areas tend to be active noisy times. Teach the children that, in this room, books go in one place, dolls in another, and blocks somewhere else. It's best, if possible, to group these noisy time areas away from your book corner and other areas such as Math, manipulatives and Science, where children need to concentrate.

2. Store materials and toys close to where they will be used by children. Children are more likely to put on a smock while playing with water, for instance, if the smocks are hung close to the water table.

3. Put messy activities over hard surface flooring for easy cleanup. Art, woodworking, water and sand play, and eating are best done over hard flooring so that spills are not a major problem.

4. Avoid having a large open space in the middle of the room. This invites children to run. Instead, use furniture and other dividers to break up the space.

5. Create smaller spaces and visual dividers between activity centers. If children can see all the other activities going on in the room they will be distracted more easily and will play with less concentration. Shelves and low dividers can be used to separate spaces visually for children but still allow adults to supervise. Such smaller spaces allow children to separate themselves from the larger group and be alone or with one or two friends—important considerations in group care situations.

6. Use the backs of shelves (used as dividers) for displays related to the activity area they are facing. This allows you to display materials at children's eye level and adds color and interest to your room. Pegboard backs can also be used to hang materials such as musical instruments or games stored in bags with handles.

SAFETY CONSIDERATIONS

1. Use quality furniture and equipment that is not likely to break under heavy use, has smooth surfaces and rounded corners, and is designed for use by children.

2. Stabilize furniture. Cubbies should be wider at the base for greater stability. Put tall or tippy shelves against the wall, back-to-back, or bolt them together in L-formations. Secure all furniture, shelves and "cubbies" so that there is absolutely no danger of equipment falling. Children tend to climb on everything and anything. Make sure all is bolted.

3. Keep traffic patterns in mind. Do not block exits.

4. Teach staff and children not to misuse equipment. Shelves are not for climbing; tables are not for standing on; blocks are not for throwing; etc. It boils down to good supervision.

5. Have several cleanup times each day so that the room does not become cluttered, leading to falls and loss or breakage of toys.

A PLANNING TOOL

It seems that some people can visualize how a room will look arranged differently and can start pushing furniture into place. If you're not one of those people—and most of us are not—you may find yourself with a sore back and a room arrangement that still doesn't work well. A less tiring way to visualize room arrangements and that allows you to experiment with no physical exertion, is to create a scaled floor plan on grid paper with scaled templates that represent your major pieces of furniture. Measure the walled spaces of your classroom and create an outline on the grid paper representing the shape of your room. Indicate where doors, windows, sink and carpeting are located. Then pick out or create templates to represent your furniture. Move these template shapes around on your floor plan until you see an arrangement you like. Contact Environments, Inc. and request their free planning grid. They also provide an extensive Early Childhood equipment and supply catalog. I have been completely satisfied with all aspects of purchasing from this company. Call toll free (800-EI-CHILD) or write to Environments, Inc., Box 1348, Beaufort Industrial Park, Beaufort, South Carolina 29901-1348. Additional phone number for Environments, Inc. is 803-846-8155.

HINTS FOR ORGANIZED
INDIVIDUAL INTEREST CENTERS:

THE HOUSEKEEPING CORNER
AND DRAMATIC PLAY AREAS

Standard pieces of equipment for the housekeeping area are a child-sized stove, sink, refrigerator, table and chairs, and doll bed. There are numerous other pieces of furniture available to enhance this area of your room, including soft living room furniture. Pots and pans, dishes, dress-up clothes, purses, etc. and, of course, dolls, are also essential for this area. There are now lovely "multi-ethnic" dolls available. Try to represent both boys and girls. Don't forget to put a shelf in this area to hold shoes, purses, boxes and other play enrichments.

See what you can do to make your "playhouse" area visually different from the rest of the room. "Kitchen" wallpaper could be put on the wall from about four feet down. Rather than having the furniture against the wall, put some of it out in the middle of the room, facing the wall, to make the outside "wall" of the "room." Consider dividing this area to make two or three rooms—a kitchen, bedroom and living room. The more elaborate you make it, the richer the play will be.

Children's cubbies should be labeled and kept neat for parents' convenience.

Also offer children frequent dramatic play opportunities in settings other than the "house" and locate them close to the housekeeping corner. "Storefront-type" pieces of equipment are available that can be used indoors or outdoors. Their uses are only limited by your imagination. A store, an office, a bank, etc., give children natural extensions for their dramatic play in the housekeeping area.

THE BLOCK AREA

Large hollow blocks can be stacked on the floor against the wall. Hinged storage shelf units are ideal for unit blocks. A hinged shelf unit opened to an L position has maximum stability and you need not put the shelf against the wall. If you have the block shelf against the wall facing the room, the blocks will tend to expand outward, often extending into the traffic pattern. It works better to put the shelf out in the middle of the room eight or ten feet from the wall and facing the corner.

Store the larger, heavier unit blocks on the bottom shelves. Trace the shapes of the blocks onto colored self-stick paper, cut these out, and stick them to the shelves where the blocks are to be stored. Accessories such as wooden people and animals, train sets and miniature traffic signs can be stored in separate bins, in compartments in the shelf or on top. It's fun to use colored plastic tape to make "parking places" on the floor against the wall for the cars and trucks.

Be sure to provide ample space in this area. If the children are cramped and cannot get to the shelves comfortably, they are more likely to knock over someone else's blocks and frustration will build. Use colored plastic tape to put a line on the floor about twelve inches out parallel to the shelf.

Teach children not to build between the line and the shelf; this allows space for other children to get to the shelf. As children will be sitting on the floor when they play here, it is good to put this activity in a carpeted area of the classroom. (Also, falling blocks make less noise on carpet!)

The block corner usually works well close to the housekeeping corner. They are both fairly "noisy," active play areas, and the materials combine well.

GROSS-MOTOR PLAY AREA

It's a good idea to have well-designed gross-motor toys indoors, such as rocking boats, well-made climbers with mats under them, and/or large vinyl-coated nylon-covered foam pieces to crawl, jump and roll on.

Perhaps you are fortunate enough to have a separate room for this. If these things are in your regular classroom, they need a lot of space for safety. Be conscious of what children can reach from the top of the climber. Be sure that light fixtures, electric cords, drapery cords and any other objects that may be dangerous are well out of reach.

Gross-motor toys usually go well near your housekeeping and dramatic play areas, often extending the play.

THE ART AREA

Design your art area for independence on the part of children. Children can be taught to put on their own smocks if they are hung where children can reach them. An open shelf should offer a changing variety of art supplies and collage materials to which children can help themselves. Can the children reach the sink comfortably? Consider adding a small step so that they can wash out their own brushes and wash their hands when they finish working. Keep a large sponge within their reach so that they can wipe up their own spills. Adjust easels so that they are at children's eye level.

A table is necessary in your art area for small group projects and independent work. Locate the art area near the sink in your room and over hard-surfaced flooring for easy cleanup of spills. Put your largest wastebasket here.

Your water/sand table should also be located over hard flooring for easy cleanup. A water/sand table has multiple uses. From time to time, change what is in it to add variety to children's sensory experiences. It could contain clay, shaving cream, birdseed, cotton balls, a cornstarch and water goo mixture and many other things. A storage shelf should be nearby to hold play materials such as plastic bottles, funnels, scoops and tubing.

THE WOODWORKING AREA

This area works well close to the art corner because children love to enhance their constructions with glue, paint, string and collage materials. Purchase a sturdy woodworking bench designed for use by children. Make sure it has a vise for holding pieces of wood steady while they are being sawed. Pegboard is ideal for storing carpentry tools. Cut an outline shape of each tool from self-stick paper and stick it to the Pegboard where the tool should go. A small broom and dustpan will encourage children to clean up. A magnet is good for picking up spilled nails. The woodworking area must be easy to supervise.

THE SCIENCE CENTER

Your science area will work well close to a window so that plants will thrive. Provide a shelf on which to store materials such as magnifying glasses, magnets, tweezers, a balance scale and sorting games. You will also need a table for display and active involvement with the materials, and a place for animal cages and an aquarium. Make sure that there is something for children to do in the science area, instead of only things to look at; otherwise, this area will not absorb its share of children and that many more of them will be competing for the other areas of your room.

THE MATH AREA

Math materials are often included in the science area or in the manipulatives area of the classroom. But in kindergarten and prekindergarten classrooms, teachers often choose to create a special math center. There are certainly many interesting things to put here, such as a balance scale, geoboards, dice and playing cards. Again, a shelf for storage and a table for play are ideal.

MANIPULATIVES AREA

The main challenge with this area, which houses "table toys" (puzzles, beads, pegs and pegboards, and construction toys with many pieces) is to prevent things from getting all mixed up and pieces getting lost. Sturdy, transparent plastic bins are ideal storage for such toys. If you put a picture of the toy on the shelf where the bin goes, putting the toys away becomes a matching activity and teaches order. Some teachers provide cafeteria trays for children to build on. This seems to help keep the pieces from spreading too far.

THE BOOKS AND LANGUAGE AREA

A good early childhood program exposes children to quantities of good children's literature. Organize books neatly on a sturdy bookshelf, so that their full fronts show, not just their spines. You will also need a shelf or table for magazines, puppets and language games. It's nice to have a felt board and materials here for children to play with. A low bulletin board or display area will allow you to post pictures that encourage children to use language and increase their vocabulary.

You need good light in this spot because children will be looking at print and illustrations. Divide this area off from the rest of the room as much as possible so that children can concentrate more easily. Make it cozy and inviting, with pillows and/or some of the wonderful soft vinyl-coated nylon-covered foam pieces now available. This area can become a place of refuge to the child who needs to get away from the bustle of the group and can be a nice place for a teacher to spend some one-on-one time with children.

THE MUSIC AREA

Rhythm instruments can be hung on a pegboard back of a shelf. Plastic streamers are a lovely addition to encourage creative movement. A record player or cassette player to provide music can also be added. Provide enough space in this area to allow children to dance and move to music. If you use colored plastic tape to create a circle on the floor, children like to dance in or on the circle. In some classrooms this activity center doubles as their group time or circle time area.

CIRCLE TIME AREA

Sometimes the language or music area is used for circle time. The space needs to be large enough for all the children in the group to sit down on the floor at one time. It is good to have this in a carpeted section of the room. An area rug can help define the space, even one placed over your regular carpeting. A low bulletin board and a wall-mounted flannel board will find good use here. Try to reduce distractions for children by having the teacher seat and focal point against a wall.

A PARENT AREA

An important part of your room is the parent communication area. Parents will look at an attractive bulletin board if you keep it changing, put up informative articles and add occasional photographs of their children at play, etc. A box with a divider in it for each child placed on a table or shelf can hold art work to take home. Children's cubbies should be labeled and kept neat for parents' convenience as well as for attractiveness. How about adding an adult-sized chair or bench so that parents can sit down as they help children with boots and snowsuits and say their good-byes in the morning?

COTS AND NAPTIME ARRANGEMENTS

If yours is an all-day program, you will need a cot or rest mat for every child in attendance. Each cot or mat should be labeled with the child's name. Cots or mats should be stored out of the way when not in use. Children's blankets must be stored so that they do not touch each other. Your state child care licensing regulations will probably require that there be a floor plan designating where each child's cot will be placed, and regulations will state how many inches between cots are required. If your space is minimal, it can sometimes be a challenge fitting all the rest cots or mats in the floor space you have available. You may have to move one or two shelves slightly to accommodate. Do not let this deter you from having a good room arrangement with furniture dividing areas. Simply make moving the few pieces of furniture a regular part of your routine.

A FINAL THOUGHT

You can tell a lot about what a teacher or day care director values by how she or he arranges and organizes the space in the center. Your center reflects you and what you think is important for children. This is a place where you and the children spend many hours—make it the best it can be.

(The preceding section is reprinted with permission from Environments, Inc.)

EQUIPMENT AND SUPPLIES

We must begin with a word of caution here: before purchasing any equipment and/or supplies, evaluate the safety considerations. Although the toy may appear safe and is advertised in a brochure, catalog or displayed at a trade show exhibit, it may not be safe or appropriate for all age groups. It is better to be safe than sorry certainly applies in all matters related to a child's health and safety.

The Educational Specialists at Environments, Inc., have an equipment and materials list to be used as a guide for classroom planning. If you have questions or would like free planning assistance, you may call them at 800-EI-CHILD, or write Environments, Inc., P.O. Box 1348, Beaufort, SC 29901.

WHERE CAN I OBTAIN FREE SUPPLIES?

Listed below are some locations where I obtained free materials that were fashioned into arts and crafts projects. The types of materials commonly available from these sources are also listed for each one. Use your knowledge and imagination to think of other supplies they may provide you with!

Wallpaper store	old sample books
Paint store	sample paint charts
Lumber yard	scraps of wood (pine is preferable), pieces of lumber—use for building blocks. (Make sure wood has not been treated with harmful chemicals.)
Carpet store	floor samples
Fabric store	spools, scraps, eyelet, ribbons, buttons
Tobacco shop	cigar boxes
Printer	paper in a variety of colors, shapes, textures
Garment factory	pieces of fabric
Label factory	stickers
Furniture and appliance stores	large boxes
Farm store	ice cream cartons
Computer centers	printout paper
Cabinet makers	wooden color samples
Medical suppliers, clinics, drug stores	tongue depressors and styrofoam
Grocery stores, liquor stores, shoe stores	boxes and containers

Post Office	ends from sheets of stamps—you can color the zip code man and on the blank ones, you can design your own stamp
Newspaper printer	end rolls (for drawing paper)
Electric supply store	thin wire
Bar or restaurant	wine corks
Airlines	plastic cups
Architectural firm	drafting paper
Billboard companies	large sheets of colored paper
Bottling companies	bottle caps
Container companies	large sheets of cardboard
Contractors	building scraps, linoleum pieces, sawdust
Power companies	telephone poles, spools
Candy manufacturers	cans and boxes
Moving company	large boxes
Gift shop	styrofoam packing pieces
Fast food outlets	plates, napkins, "freebies," empty sour cream and margarine containers, etc.
Tire store	truck or tractor tires for climbing

WHAT PARENTS CAN SAVE

"One man's junk is another's treasure." No truer words were ever spoken especially in projects involving children. The odd items we throw away without thought can provide creative and pleasurable hours of activities for children. Ask the parents to keep a box or bag in a cabinet. Children are thrilled to issue reminders to their parents about saving a paper towel roll or margarine container. It is another area of "school-life" that the child and parent can share.

Here's a mini-list. You are bound to think of other items you can use.

margarine containers	plastic lids of all sizes
empty oatmeal containers	old magazines and catalogs
baby food jars	egg cartons
light-weight cardboard	shirt cardboards
cardboard rolls from paper towels, foil and plastic wrap	junk mail
toilet paper rolls	spring-type clothespins
pipe cleaners	straws
tin cans with plastic lids	brown paper bags
clean, old clothes	frozen juice cans
large boxes	used paper cups
long shoelaces	shoe boxes
1/2 gallon milk or juice containers	heavy string
old calendars	tin foil
old greeting cards	paper plates
ribbon, yarn	construction paper
pinecones	wrapping paper scraps
masking tape	old toothbrushes
hard white beans	old tractor tires
deck of cards (full or partial)	corn kernels
ping pong balls	large paint brushes
	cotton balls
	fabric scraps

My favorite sources of free supplies are retail stores, fast food restaurants, supermarkets, video stores, etc. As you walk through malls, supermarkets and shopping centers, note the decorations and product cartons that are displayed. For example, I approach the managers of Hallmark Greeting Card Stores and ask them to save their holiday decorations for my day care bulletin boards. I call after every season. Supermarkets have given me cardboard-house cookie displays. Video stores have passed along Walt Disney-type posters. Just look around and don't be afraid to ask stores to save. Many proprietors like to "unload" seasonal decorations after a promotion. Don't worry if they say "no" to your request. They just may say "yes"... and after all, it's free!

TOOLBOX TIPS

When you actually sit down to design your advertising brochure, flyer, etc. you may wonder what to say. Perhaps some of the words and phrases below will help. Experiment by combining some of the following:

For Friendly Beginnings

New Infant Program

Accredited by the National Academy of Early Childhood Programs

Computers, Trips, Fenced Yard...

State Licensed

Licensed by PA Dept. of Education & Welfare

Affectionate, Understanding Staff

Registered Nurse

Announcing a New Addition!

Finest Day Camp

Now Accepting Applications

Open House

FREE Week

New Extended Hours

Register NOW!

Small Classes

Before & After School Drop-Ins

Come & See!

Educational Programs

Field Trips, Crafts, Gymnastics

Opening in June, Enrolling Now!

Limited Openings

Focus on Positive Self-Esteem

Science and Nature Activities

Music, Art & Drama Experiences

Special Transportation Available

Care for Sick Children

Experienced, Degreed Teachers

Loving Environment

Year Round Programs

High Quality Program

Celebrating 25 Years in Education

APPENDIX 1

CURRENT STATE DAY CARE LICENSING OFFICES

Child care programs are regulated by each state and subject to change. Most states specify the minimum requirements. In order to provide a quality, self-sustaining profitable business, you will need to exceed what is mandated. In order to find out the standards you must meet, contact the appropriate office listed below. If you send $1 and a self-addressed stamped envelope to the Child Care Action Campaign, you will receive a list of the most current addresses (CCAC, 330 Seventh Ave., 17th Floor, New York, NY 10001). In addition, contact the local Resource and Referral service for detailed information and training for programs in your area. R&R's, as they are called, help parents find child care by maintaining a database of licensed caregivers. They also recruit and train new child care providers. The R&R in your area is probably listed in the Yellow Pages under "Child Care."

In each state, there are three types of contacts—Child Care Licensing Official, Advocacy Contact and Title XX Child Care Administrator.

Alabama Dept. of Human Resources
50 North Ripley Street
Montgomery, Alabama 36130
(205) 261-5360

Dept. of Health & Social Services
Division of Family & Youth Services
230 South Franklin St., Suite 206
Juneau, Alaska 99801
(907) 465-3013

Arizona Dept. of Health Services
Office of Children
Day Care Facilities Division
100 West Clerdon St., 4th floor
Phoenix, Arizona 85013
(602) 255- 1272

Division of Children & Family Services
Child Care Licensing Office,
Room 607
Day Care Licensing Division
P.O. Box 1437
Little Rock, Arkansas 72203
(501) 682-8590

Community Care Licensing
Dept. of Social Services,
Day Care Unit
744 P Street, Mail Station 19-50
Sacramento, California 95814
(916) 324-4031

Department of Social Services
Day Care Unit
605 Bannock Street, Room 354
Denver, Colorado 80204
(303) 893-7166

Community Nursing Home Health Div.
Child Day Care Licensing Unit
141150 Washington Street
Hartford, Connecticut 06106
(203) 566-2575

Licensing Bureau
Delaware Youth and Family Center
1825 Faulkland Road
Wilmington, Delaware 19805
(302) 633-2695

Licensing & Certification Division
Social Services Branch
614 H Street, NW, Room 1031
Washington, D.C. 20001
(202) 727-7226

Office of Children, Youth & Families
Dept. of Health and Rehab. Services
1317 Winewood Blvd.
Tallahassee, Florida 32399
(904) 488-4900

Child Care Licensing Office, Room 607
Department of Human Resources
878 Peachtree Street, N.E.
Atlanta, Georgia 30309
(404) 894-5688

Division of Social Services
P.O. Box 2816
Agana, Guam 96910
011 (671) 734-7399

Department of Human Services,
Licensing Unit
420 Weiaka Milo Road, Suite 101
Honolulu, Hawaii 96817-4941
(808) 832-5025

Department of Health & Welfare
Family and Children's Division
4355 Emerald Street, 2nd floor
Boise, Idaho 83706
(208) 334-6800

Dept. of Children & Family Services
406 East Monroe Avenue
Springfield, Illinois 62701-1498
(217) 785-2598

State of Indiana,
Dept. of Public Welfare
Child Welfare/Social Service Division
402 West Washington St,. Rm. W364
Indianapolis, Indiana 46204
(317) 232-4440

Division of Adult, Children
& Family Services
Iowa Department of Human Services
Hoover State Office Building
Des Moines, Iowa 50319
(515) 281-6074

Kansas Dept. of Health & Environment
Landon State Office Bldg.
Child Care Lic. Section
900 S.W. Jackson Street
Topeka, Kansas 66612-1290
(913) 296-1275

Division of Licensing and Regulation
Cabinet for Human Resources Building
Fourth Floor East
Frankfort, Kentucky 40621
(502) 564-2800

Dept. of Social Services
Dept. of Health & Hospitals
P.O. Box 3767/P.O. Box 3078
Baton Rouge, Louisiana 70821
(504) 342-6446

Department of Human Services
Bureau of Child & Family Services
221 State Street
Augusta, Maine 04333
(207) 289-5060

Office of Licensing and Certification
Division of Child Care Centers
4201 Patterson Avenue
Baltimore, Maryland 21215
(301) 764-2750

Office for Children
10 West Street
Boston, Massachusetts 02111
(617) 727-8956

Division of Child Day Care Licensing
Michigan Dept. of Social Services
235 South Grand Street, Suite 1212
P.O. Box 30037
Lansing, Michigan 48909
(517) 373-8300

Department of Human Services
Division of Licensing
444 Lafayette Road
St. Paul, Minnesota 55155-3842
(612) 296-3971

Division of Child Care &
Special Licensure
Mississippi State Department of Health
P.O. Box 1700
Jackson, Mississippi 39215-1700
(601) 960-7504

State Department of Social Services
Div. of Family Services
State Office of Child Care
Licensing Unit
P.O. Box 88
Jefferson City, Missouri 65103
(314) 751-2450

Department of Family Services
P.O. Box 8005
Helena, Montana 59604
(406) 444-5900

Department of Social Services
P.O. Box 95026
301 Centennial Mall South, 5th floor
Lincoln, Nebraska 68509-5062
(402) 471-3121

Bureau of Services for Child Care
505 East King St., Rm. 101
Carson City, Nevada 89710
(702) 687-5911

Division of Public Health Services
Bureau of Child Care Standards & Lic.
Health & Human Services Building
6 Hazen Drive
Concord, New Hampshire 03301
(603) 271-4624

Bureau of Licensing
Div. of Youth & Family Services
CN 717
Trenton, New Jersey 08625-0717
(609) 292-9220

Licensing Health-Related Facilities
Public Health Division
1190 St. Francis Drive
Santa Fe, New Mexico 87503
(505) 827-2389

Bureau of Day Care Licensing
Mississippi State Department of Health
65 Worth St., 4th floor
P.O. Box 1700
New York, New York 10013

N.Y. State Dept. of Social Services
40 North Pearl St.
Albany, New York 12243
(800) 342-3715

Office of Child Day Care Licensing
Child Day Care Section
701 Barbour Drive
Raleigh, North Carolina 27603
(919) 733-4801

North Dakota Dept. of Human Services
Children & Family Services Division
Judicial Wing, 3rd floor
600 East Boulevard Avenue
Bismarck, North Dakota 58505-0250
(701) 224-3580

Office of Child Care Services
30 East Broad Street, 30th floor
Columbus, Ohio 43266-0423
(614) 466-3822

Department of Human Services
Child Care Licensing Unit
P.O. Box 25352
Oklahoma City, Oklahoma 73125
(405) 521-3561

Department of Human Resources
Children's Services Division
198 Commercial Street, S.E.
Salem, Oregon 97310
(503) 378-3178

Pennsylvania Dept. of Public Welfare
Central Region Day Care Services
P.O. Box 2675
Lanco Lodge Building 25
Harrisburg, Pennsylvania 17105
(717) 787-8691

Department of Social Services
Family Services Secretary
P.O. Box 11398
Fernandez Juncos Station
Santurce, Puerto Rico 00910
(809) 723-2127

Department of Children &
Their Families
Day Care Licensing Unit
610 Mount Pleasant Ave., Building 2
Providence, Rhode Island 02908
(401) 457-4708

South Carolina Dept. of Social Services
Day Care Licensing Division
P.O. Box 1520
Columbia, South Carolina 29202-1520
(803) 734-5740

Department of Social Services
Child Protection Services
Richard F. Kneip Building
700 Governor's Drive
Pierre, South Dakota 57501-2291
(605) 773-3227

Day Care Licensing Division
Tennessee Dept. of Human Services
1000 Second Avenue
P.O. Box 1135
Nashville, Tennessee 37202
(615) 244-9706

Texas Dept. of Human Services
Day Care Licensing Division
P.O. Box 149030, W-403
Austin, Texas 78714-9030
(512) 450-3261

Division of Human Services,
Office of Licensing
120 North, 200 West
Salt Lake City, Utah 84145
(801) 538-4242

Licensing & Regulations Division,
Day Care Unit
Dept. of Social & Rehab. Services
103 South Main Street
Waterbury, Vermont 05676
(802) 241-2158

Department of Human Services
Barbel Plaza South
St. Thomas, Virgin Islands 00801
(809) 774-9030

Division of Licensing Programs
Department of Social Services, Ste. 219
8007 Discovery Drive, Tyler Bldg.
Richmond, Virginia 23239
(804) 662-9025

Dept. of Social & Health Services
Div. of Children & Family Services
P.O. Box 45710
Olympia, Washington 98504
(206) 586-2688

West Virginia Dept. of
Human Resources
Office of Social Services
Building 6, Room 850
Charleston, West Virginia 25305
(304) 348-7980

Day Care Licensing
Department of Health and
Social Services
3601 Memorial Drive
Madison, Wisconsin 53704
(608) 249-0441

Division of Public Assistance
& Social Services
Family Services Unit
Hathaway Building, 3rd Floor
Cheyenne, Wyoming 82002

Child Care Action Campaign
330 Seventh Avenue, 17th Floor
New York, New York 10001
(212) 239-0138

APPENDIX 2

CHILD CARE ORGANIZATIONS

This list is not intended to be a comprehensive account of all child care resources and programs. The following organizations may be useful for additional information on work, family and child care issues. Explore all sources of information pertinent to your intended program. Ask the national associations for information about local affiliated groups for your networking purposes.

Child Care Employee Project
6536 Telegraph Ave., Suite A201
Oakland, CA 94609
(510) 653-9889
A clearinghouse on child care employee issues such as salaries, status and working conditions. Publishes a newsletter, *CHILD CARE EMPLOYEE NEWS*, and offers membership. It is the national resource clearinghouse on child care staffing issues as well as a leader in advocating for better regulations and funding of child care services.

National Association of Hospital Affiliated Child Care Programs
Shawnee Mission Medical Center
Child Care Center
9100 West 74th St.
Overland Park, KS 66210
Members of the NAHACCP receive a list of hospital affiliated child care programs, a newsletter and participation in the annual conference.

Council for Early Childhood Professional Recognition
1341 G St. NW
Suite 400
Washington, DC 20005-3105
(800) 424-4310
(202) 265-9090
Administers a nationally recognized credentialing program for caregivers. Awards the Child Development Associate Credential (CDA). In some states, an individual needs only a CDA credential to qualify for a director or teacher position. In other states, this individual would need to verify additional education and/or experience. Each state has the power to establish qualifications for staff who work in licensed child care centers.

Child Welfare League of America
440 First St. NW
Washington, DC 20001-2085
(202) 638-2952

Coalition of Labor Union Women
15 Union Square
New York, NY 10011
(212) 242-0700

National Women's Law Center
1616 P St. NW
Washington, DC 20036
(202) 328-5160

Parent Action
2 Hopkins Plaza, Suite 2100
Baltimore, MD 21201
(410) 752-1790

Work and Family Clearinghouse
U.S. Department of Labor
Women's Bureau
200 Constitution Ave. NW
Washington, DC 20005
(800) 827-5335
(202) 219-4486

Families and Work Institute
330 Seventh Ave., 14th Floor
New York, NY 10001
(212) 465-2044

Families USA
1334 G St. NW, 3rd Floor
Washington, DC 20005
(202) 737-6340

The Children's Defense Fund
122 E St. NW
Washington, DC 20001
(202) 628-8787
Annually publishes the *State Child Care Fact Book* which summarizes the child care public policy in each state, including programs and funding levels. Subscription newsletter available, CDF Reports.

National Association for the Education of Young Children
1509 Sixteenth St. NW
Washington, D.C. 20036
(800) 424-2460
Largest professional group of early childhood educators/child care providers. Publishes the journal *YOUNG CHILDREN*, brochures, posters, videotapes and books. National, state, and local affiliate groups offer training opportunities and networking meetings. The Information Services Group is very helpful as a resource.

National Black Child Development Institute
1023 15th St. NW
Suite 600
Washington, DC 20005
(202) 387-1281
Publishes a newsletter, *THE BLACK CHILD ADVOCATE*, and calendar featuring issues and important dates in history relevant to the development of black children. Membership, conferences, resource catalog.

The Child Care Action Campaign
330 Seventh Ave., 17th Floor
New York, NY 10001
(212) 239-0138
A national not-for-profit advocacy membership organization that supports programs that will increase the availability of quality, affordable child care for the nation. Provides information to parents, providers, leaders from corporations and labor, the media, government and community. The campaign's board members are CEO's of a number of Fortune 500 companies, editors-in-chief of national magazines, academicians and heads of major child advocacy organizations. Newsletter and membership. Contact them for timely reports on the issue of child care.

The Children's Foundation
725 15th St. NW, Suite 505
Washington, DC 20005
(202) 347-3300

The National Association for Family Day Care
1331 Pennsylvania Ave., Suite 548
Washington, DC 20004
(800) 359-3817

Child Care Food Program
U.S. Department of Agriculture
Washington, DC 20250
Sponsors nutrition education and reimburses partial and full food costs for some child care

programs. Contact the local licensing office to find sponsors for your area. The Child and Adult Care Food Program (CACFP) is a federal program whose primary focus is to improve the diet of children and adults in licensed and approved non-profit organizations. Certain food groups and portions are specified to be served in order to qualify for financial assistance.

Cooperative Extensive Service Located in local county government offices. Free and inexpensive material on child care, child development and other topics of interest to providers. Look in the white pages of your phone book under your county's name. (For example: Bucks County Government-Cooperative Extensive Service.) May also be associated with your state LAND GRANT university. In Pennsylvania, that is Penn State University.

National Association for Clinical Infant Programs
2000 14th St. North, Suite 380
Arlington, VA 22201-2500
(703) 528-4300
Publishes information and sponsors conferences on infant health, mental health and development.

National Association of Child Care Resource and Referral Agencies
Box 40246
Washington, DC 20016-0246
(202) 393-5501
Can provide information on child care initiatives, training programs and local child care resources.

Association of Child Care Consultants International
109 S. Bloodworth St.
Raleigh, NC 27601
(919) 834-6506
Goals are to maintain the highest possible professional standards within the field, to provide

leadership and to provide a network for the interaction of consultants for professional support and development. The Child Care Action Campaign sells a publication, *AN EMPLOYER'S GUIDE TO CHILD CARE CONSULTANTS*, which focuses on: the reasons for using a consultant, services that consultants can offer, how to choose a child care consultant and resources for locating child care consultants.

School-Age Child Care Project
Wellesley College
Center for Research on Women
Wellesley, MA 02181
(617) 283-2500
Clearinghouse on school-age programs, latchkey children issues. Newsletter.

ERIC Clearinghouse on Elementary and Early Childhood Education (ERIC/EECE)
College of Education
University of Illinois
805 W. Pennsylvania Ave.
Urbana, IL 61801-4877
(217) 333-1386
Computer searches on any early childhood topic. Ask your librarian for more information. Contact for complete description of valuable services.

American Academy of Pediatrics
Box 927
141 Northwest Point Blvd.
Elk Grove Village, IL 60009
(708) 228-5005
(800) 433-9016
Publications available: 1. *HEALTH IN DAY CARE: A MANUAL FOR HEALTH PROFESSIONALS*; 2. *CARING FOR OUR CHILDREN- NATIONAL HEALTH AND SAFETY PERFORMANCE STANDARDS: GUIDELINES FOR OUT-OF-HOME CHILD CARE PROGRAMS* (American Academy of Pediatrics/American Public Health Association)—this book discusses recommended

diaper standards to prevent the spread of infectious diseases in day care environments as well as many other health and safety concerns.

The Center for Early Adolescence
3 to 6 p.m. Project
University of North Carolina at Chapel Hill
D 2 Carr Mill Town Center
Carrboro, NC 27510
(919) 966-1148
Offers curriculum catalog of programs found to be exemplary for out-of-school, after hours child care. Training materials for caregivers to meet the needs of early adolescence.

New York State School of Industrial and Labor Relations
Cornell University
Ives Hall, Room 194
Ithaca, NY 14851-0952
ILR REPORT: WORKING PARENTS, published twice a year.

Phone Friend
Box 735
State College, PA 16804
Information on setting up telephone hotlines, warm lines for children staying home alone after school.

The Conference Board
845 Third Ave.
New York, NY 10022
(212) 759-0900

Work/Family Directions, Inc.
930 Commonwealth Ave. South
Boston, MA 02215-1212
(617) 278-4000
Child and Elder Care consulting firm. Resource and referrals.

American Medical Association
515 N. State St.
Chicago, IL 60610
(312) 464-5000

National Child Care Association
1029 Railroad St.
Conyers, GA 30207
(800) 543-7161
An alliance of proprietary child care providers.

The Center for the Study of Public Policies for Young Children
High/Scope Education Research Foundation
600 North River St.
Ypsilanti, MI 48198
(313) 485-2000

Bank Street College of Education
610 West 112th St.
New York, NY 10025
(212) 875-4400

Family Resource Coalition
230 North Michigan Ave.,
Suite 1625
Chicago, IL 60601
(312) 341-0900

Wheelock College
200 The Riverway
Boston, MA 02215
(617) 734-5200

Catalyst
250 Park Ave. South
New York, NY 10003-1459
(212) 239-0138
Offers a resource guide, *RESOURCES FOR TODAY'S PARENTS*, which lists organizations, publications, videos, etc., on a variety of topics related to child care and parenting.

Employee Benefits Research Institute
2121 K St. NW
Suite 600
Washington, DC 20037
(202) 775-6300

Employees Council on Flexible Compensation
927 15th St. NW, Suite 1000
Washington, DC 20005
(202) 659-4300

National Council of Jewish Women
Center for the Child
53 W. 23rd St.
New York, NY 10010
(212) 645-4048

New Ways to Work
149 Ninth St.
San Francisco, CA 94103
(415) 553-1000

Regional Research Institute for
Human Services
Portland State University
Box 751
Portland, OR 97267

Resources for Child Care
Management
261 Springfield Ave., Suite 201
Berkeley Heights, NJ 07922
(908) 665-9070

U.S. General Accounting Office
Box 6015
Gaithersburg, MD 20877
The Superintendent of Documents
offers a free copy of *CHILD CARE:
EMPLOYER ASSISTANCE FOR
PRIVATE SECTOR AND FEDERAL
EMPLOYEES*. Discusses and defines
the various options. Examines the
costs, benefits, advantages and
disadvantages of on-site, voucher
and vendor child care, consortium
and on-site child care programs.
Send a postcard request.

U.S.Department of Labor
Women's Bureau
200 Constitution Ave. NW
Washington, DC 20210
(202) 219-6611
Offers a free pamphlet, *Employers
and Child Care: Establishing Services
Through the Workplace*. Provides
guidance for on-site and family day
care programs.

9 to 5
National Association
of Working Women
614 Superior Ave. NW
Cleveland, OH 44113

Institute for Child Care
Professionals
Box 682286
Houston, TX 77268-2286
Presents management seminars
addressing leadership, effective
supervision, decision making
and time-management for child
care directors.

APPENDIX 3

EXAMPLES OF EMPLOYER SPONSORED CHILD CARE PROGRAMS

Companies and employers sponsor a variety of child care programs for their employees including: on-site or near-site care, family day care network, child care reimbursement program, child care voucher program and dependent care spending account, financial assistance, information referral and assistance for regular care and sick care, transportation between centers and subsidies.

Before opening an employer-sponsored child care center, read current literature, visit centers and learn from the experiences of others.

ON OR NEAR-SITE CENTERS:
Merck Pharmaceuticals - Rahway, New Jersey and West Point, Pennsylvania
The Stride-Rite Foundation - Boston, Massachusetts
Bowles Corporation - North Ferrisburg, Vermont
Chalet Dental Clinic - Yakima, Washington
The Cardiac Pacemakers Center - St. Paul, Minnesota
The Trammel Crow Early Learning Center - Dallas, Texas
Paramount Studios - Los Angeles, California
Johnson & Johnson- New Brunswick, New Jersey
Chrysler Corporation, United Auto Workers - Huntsville, Alabama

UNION-SPONSORED PROGRAMS:
For information on union-sponsored programs, contact AFSCME, 1625 L Street NW, Washington, DC 20036-5687 (202-429-5090). If you are a member of their organization, they will send one free copy of a list of AFSCME child care programs currently in operation. They will provide a wealth of information on many issues and options for child care operations, ONLY if you are a member of their organization.

Helpful publications *available for union members only* include:
A Labor of Love: AFSCME Child Care Examples
AFL-CIO
815 16th St. NW
Washington, DC 20006
(202) 637-5000
This is only available for union-sponsored child care programs.
If you are a member of AFSCME (American Federation of State, County and
Municipal Employees, AFL-CIO) the Women's Rights Department can
assist you with suggested reading and videos that are useful for organizing
child care campaigns and community action programs for unions. AFSCME
participates in over fifty on-site child care centers nationwide.

Putting Families First: Working Family Resource Guide
AFL-CIO
815 16th St. NW
Washington, DC 20006
(202) 637-5208
Write for price and availability of guide—only available for affiliates of
AFL-CIO union-sponsored centers.

Bargaining for Child Care: Contract Language for Union Parents
Coalition of Union Women
15 Union Square
New York, NY 10003
(212) 242-0700

ON-SITE OR NEAR-SITE CENTERS, UNION INVOLVEMENT
The Amalgamated Clothing and Textile Workers Union (ACTWU)
and Grieco Brothers, Lawrence, Massachusetts.

The American Postal Workers Union (APWU)
and U.S. Postal Service, Syracuse, New York.

The American Federation of State, County and Municipal Employees
(AFSCME) and City of Honolulu, Honolulu, Hawaii.

HOSPITAL AFFILIATED CHILD CARE PROGRAMS:
Shawnee Mission Medical Center - Overland Park, Kansas
Lutheran General Hospital - Des Plaines, Illinois
Doylestown Hospital - Doylestown, Pennsylvania
Fox Chase Medical Center - Rockledge, Pennsylvania
Pendleton Memorial Hospital - New Orleans, Louisiana
St. Mary's Hospital - Richmond, Virginia
Huntsville Hospital - Huntsville, Alabama
Northside Hospital - Atlanta, Georgia
Christian Hospital - St. Louis, Missouri
Methodist Hospital - Lubbock, Texas
Union Hospital - Terre Haute, Indiana
DC General Hospital - Washington, D.C.
Toledo Medical College - Toledo, Ohio

ADDITIONAL INFORMATION SOURCES:

Contact the Child Care Action Campaign to purchase inexpensive information guides on Employer Supported Child Care and a variety of other important summary booklets including: *Child Care Legislation, Union Involvement in Child Care, Wages and Benefits in Child Care, Sick Child Care Services, Federal Child Care Tax Credit* and up-to-date research reports. Request their publications list from:

CCAC
330 Seventh Ave., 17th Floor
New York, NY 10001
(212) 239-0138

Additional available publications and their sources are listed below:

Investing in Quality Child Care: A Report for AT&T
Mary Callery
Mail Stop
6117F3 AT5 N. Maple Ave.
Basking Ridge, NJ 07920

Options for the 90's: Employer Support for Child Care
National Council of Jewish Women
53 West 23rd St.
New York, NY 10010

Speaking with Your Employer About Child Care Assistance
Child Care Action Campaign
330 Seventh Ave., 17th Floor
New York, NY 10001
(212) 239-0138

The Employers Guide to Child Care: Developing Programs for Working Parents
Greenwood Press
88 Post Road West
Box 5007
Westport, CT 06881

Family-Supportive Policies: The Corporate Decision-Making Process
The Conference Board
845 Third Ave.
New York, NY 10022

JOINT VENTURES OR CONSORTIUM CENTERS:
Garment Industry, and the City of New York, Chinatown, New York
Communication Workers of America and U.S. West, Tempe, Arizona
Prospect Hill Office Park, Waltham, Massachusetts

APPENDIX 4

OTHER SOURCES OF HELP

U.S. Consumer Product Safety
Commission Hotline
Office of the Secretary
Washington, D.C. 20207
(800) 638-2772
Ask for guidelines for playground
equipment.

Government Printing Office
Superintendent of Documents
Publication Services
Washington, D.C. 20401
(202) 275-3050

House Document Room
H-226 Capitol
Washington, DC 20515
(202) 225-3456
Information on federal child care
bills.

Senate Document Room
Hart Office Building
Washington, DC 20515
(202) 224-7860
Information on child care
legislation.

U.S. Small Business Administration
(SBA)
Washington, DC
(800) 827-5722
This agency provides assistance in
start-up and operation of small
businesses. There are over one
hundred SBA offices nationwide.
They provide counseling,
brochures, pamphlets and seminars
for no fee or modest cost. When
you call, they have recorded
messages on financing,
management issues, starting a
business, etc. Ask for an operator
on the Small Business Desk to
answer specific questions.

Some of the other services available
through the SBA are: Small
Business Development Centers
(SBDC), the Service Corp. of Retired
Executives (SCORE), the Small
Business Institute (SBI). Each of
these groups provides counseling
and training to small businesses.

American Women's Economic
Development Corporation (AWED)
71 Vanderbilt Ave., Suite 320
New York, NY 10169
(800) 222-AWED
(212) 692-9100

National Association for
the Self-Employed
Box 612067
Dallas, TX 75261
(800) 232-NASE

Institute of Management
Accountants
10 Paragon Dr.
Montvail, NJ 07645
(800) 638-4427

National Association of Women
Business Owners
600 S. Federal St., Suite 400
Chicago, IL 60605
(312) 922-0465

National Chamber of Commerce
for Women
Ten Waterside Plaza, Suite 6H
New York, NY 10010
(212) 685-3454

Behind Small Business (newsletter)
Box 37147
Minneapolis, MN 55431

National Home Business Report
Barbara Brabec Productions
Box 2137
Naperville, IL 60565
Great ideas for all types of
businesses, including day care
centers. Subscription available.

Worksteader News (newsletter)
Box 820
Rancho Cordova, CA 95741

Other sources of help can be found in public and college libraries, State
Economic Development Agencies, Chamber of Commerce, local college
MBA offices and associations which sponsor business meetings, luncheons
and seminars.

FAMILY DAY CARE NETWORKS

Home child care providers are trained to care for the children of
employees. Employees are referred to these strictly monitored homes
through a resource and referral service.

National Treasury Employees Union and the IRS are participating
jointly in this program.

The Planning Council of Norfolk, Virginia monitors and approves
family day care homes for employees of member companies.

Chase Manhattan Bank, Con Edison, Manufacturers Hanover Bank and
American Express have provided funds to develop family day care
networks in New York City. Program operated by Child Care, Inc., a
resource and referral agency.

APPENDIX 5

JOURNALS, MAGAZINES, BOOKS AND NEWSLETTERS

Pre K Today
Scholastic Inc.
730 Broadway
New York, NY 10003
(800) 631-1586
This magazine is filled with ideas for teaching and caring for infants to five-year-olds. Subscription available.

Totline Newsletter
Warren Publishing House, Inc.
Box 2255
Everett, WA 98203
Full of creative and challenging ideas for preschool children. Subscription available.

School Age Notes
Box 120674
Nashville, Tennessee 37212
Bimonthly newsletter for providers who work with elementary school children.

No Time To Waste: An Action Agenda for School-Age Child Care
School Age Child Care Project
Wellesley College
Center for Research on Women
Wellesley, MA 02181

School-Age Child Care: An Action Manual
Auburn Publishing Company
Boston, MA

The Kids' After School Activity Book
David S. Lake Publishers
Box 741-8174
Belmont, CA 94002

Child Care Information Exchange
Box 2890
Redmond, WA 98073
(206) 883-9394
This magazine is full of useful and interesting information for day care personnel. Also offers child care director and owner seminars and conferences.

Redleaf Press
450 North Syndicate, Suite 5
Saint Paul, MN 55104-4125
(800) 423-8309
Catalog of resources, books and publications for child care providers.

Early Childhood News
330 Progress Rd.
Dayton, OH 45449
Trade publication that offers the latest innovations to make your job easier and your center more successful.

Exploring Books
Warren Publishing House, Inc.
Box 2250
Everett, WA 98203
Newsletter reviews literature for children. (Subscription)

The following books are available from NAEYC. To request a catalog or to place orders, call 800-424-2460.

Accreditation Criteria and Procedures of the National Academy of Early Childhood Programs, S. Bredecamp

Activities for School-Age Child Care, B. Blakely

Administering Programs for Young Children, J.F.Brown

Careers with Young Children: Making Your Decision, J.W. Seaver

Caring Communities: Supporting Young Children and Families

Caring: Supporting Children's Growth, R.M. Warren

The Case for Mixed-Age Grouping in Early Childhood Education, L. Katz

Congregations and Child Care: A Self Study for Churches and Synagogues and Their Early Childhood Programs

Child Care and Ill Children and Healthy Child Care Practices

Employer-Assisted Child Care Resource Guide and Information Kit on Employer-Assisted Child Care

Child Care Center and Ill Children Resource Guide

Legal Issues In Early Childhood Centers
Child Development Designs Inc.
3375 Buckingham Trail
West Bloomfield, MI 48033
Answers many of today's pressing legal questions. Priced at $7.50 per copy, it's a small investment compared to a legal consultation having an easily avoidable solution. Situations covered include: Records and Right to Privacy, Medical Care, Custody, Child Abuse and Neglect, Handicapped Children, Insurance, Contracts, Liability and more.

Parent-ing Information News
2399 Rolandale
West Bloomfield, MI 48324
Provides ready-to-use plan and the materials necessary to keep your parents active with your program. Supports the center director with new materials and ideas. Monthly. Subscription available. For orders and info call (313) 363-5030.

APPENDIX 6

OTHER SOURCES OF BOOKS AND INFORMATION

Free Money For Day Care,
Laurie Blum
Simon & Schuster
1230 Avenue of the Americas
New York, NY 10020
How to apply for start-up money
from foundations, corporations
and other funding sources.

Money Sources For Small Businesses,
William Alarid
Puma Publishing Company
1670 Coral Dr., Suite R
Santa Maria, CA 93454
How you can find private, federal,
state and corporate financing.

*Make It Yours! How To Own Your
Own Business,* Louis Muccioli
John Wiley & Sons, Inc.
605 Third Ave.
New York, NY 10158-0012
Tips on dealing with accountants,
lawyers, insurance brokers, bankers
and other professionals.

Managing the Day Care Dollars,
Gwen Morgan
Gryphon House
Box 275
Mount Ranier, MD 20822

Day Care Personnel Management
Save the Children
1447 Peachtree St. NE
Suite 700
Atlanta, GA 30309
(404) 885-1578

*A Handbook for Day Care Board
Members*
Day Care Council of New York, Inc.
22 West 38th St.
New York, NY 10018

*Start Your Own At-Home Child Care
Business* (Doubleday)
Patricia Gallagher
Box 555
Worcester, PA 19490
(215) 364-1945
($15.50)
A book that would be extremely
helpful for both day care centers
and day care homes. Provides
excellent information on:
advertising and promoting your
business, gathering the right
equipment and toys, suggested
daily activity plans, policies for
payments and other practical
matters.

*How To Entertain Children at Home
or in Preschool* (Young Sparrow
Press)
Patricia Gallagher
Box 555
Worcester, PA 19490
(215) 364-1945
($15.50)
Hundreds of creative things to do
and craft ideas for rainy day or any
day. Easy-to-do fun projects, simple
games, party treats, no-bake
cooking, finger plays and learning
activities that use simple household

materials. The book is chock full of creative ideas. It will show you what to do when a child exclaims, "but there is nothing to do!"

Raising Happy Kids on a Reasonable Budget (Betterway Books)
Patricia Gallagher
Box 555
Worcester, PA 19490
(215) 364-1945
($14.95)
Book loaded with advice on inexpensive ways to feed a family, money-saving educational tips, thrifty advice on prescriptions and healthcare, low-cost family vacations, etc. Practical advice on car maintenance, decorating for less, saving on utilities, and much more. The help in this book makes it well worth the price tag. Consider it "essential spending for your future!"

For All The Write Reasons! Forty Successful Authors, Publishers, Agents and Writers Tell You How To Get Your Book Published (Young Sparrow Press)
Patricia Gallagher
Box 555
Worcester, PA 19490
(215) 364-1945
($24.95)
If you like to write and wonder how to go about getting your book or magazine article published, this is the book you need to be successful. Patricia Gallagher and thirty-nine other experts in their field offer advice on how to: find an interested editor, agent or publisher, negotiate a favorable contract, obtain favorable book reviews, have your book mentioned in newspapers and magazines, appear on local and national television shows, and much more.

SPECIAL REPORTS FOR CAREGIVERS

Valuable idea-filled special reports detailing indoor and outdoor activities—highly recommended ($3 EACH). Permission is granted to reproduce the following three special reports for your teachers and day care staff. Great to photocopy for teacher training or staff meetings. Available for purchase by sending $3 for each report to Child Care, Box 555, Worcester, PA 19490.

1. *COOK UP SOME FUN WITH THE KIDS* - easy to make, no-cook baking ideas.

2. *NATURE AND MORE ... LET'S EXPLORE* - outdoor activities using seeds, rocks, gardens, leaves, etc.

3. *GET UP AND GO WITH YOUR KIDS* - low cost, no-cost places to go and things to do with children of all ages.

NO-COST ITEMS

ERIC – The Educational Resources Information Center is a national education information network designed to provide users with ready access to an extensive body of education-related literature. Established in 1966, ERIC is supported by the U.S. Department of Education, Office of Educational Research and Improvement.
ERIC Digests are concise reports on timely issues. Up to five Digests may be requested per order.
ERIC Clearinghouse on Elementary and Early Childhood Education
University of Illinois
805 W. Pennsylvania Ave.
Urbana, IL 61801-4897
(217) 333-1386
Titles available:
Multiple Perspectives on the Quality of Early Childhood Programs, by Lilian G. Katz
Having Friends, Making Friends, and Keeping Friends: Relationships as Educational Contexts, by Willard W. Hartup
Teacher-Parent Partnerships, by Kevin J. Swick
Aggression and Cooperation: Helping Young Children Develop Constructive Strategies, by Jan Jewett

APPENDIX 7

CURRICULUM PLANNING KITS
Kapers for Kids
2325 Endicott St.
St. Paul, MN 55114
(800) 882-7332
The Kapers for Kids monthly
curriculum program includes a
sixty-page curriculum guide with
teaching units, music booklet,
special day activities, cassette sing-
a-long tape, flannelboard pictures,
activity booklets for each child,
crafts with materials for each
child, etc.

Little People's Workshop
Box 43900
Louisville, KY 40253
(800) 626-1554
Step-by-step learning activities to
stimulate children. Lessons for
circle time, art, movement and
so on.

VIDEOS
Write for price, availability and
ordering information.

*Child Care Challenge: Union
Solutions*
LIPA (Labor Institute Public Affairs)
815 16th St., Suite 206
Washington, DC 20006
(202) 637-5334

*Quality Child Care: It's a
Business Issue*
Child Care American Video
Box 5010
Ronkonkuma, NY 11779

AUDIO TAPES
Julie Wassom
The Julian Group
Box 61458
Denver, Colorado 80206
1-800-876-0260
*Employers as Prospects: The Provider's
Guide to Marketing and Selling
Employer Sponsored Child Care
Programs:* An invaluable resource
guide of strategies, approaches and
systems for successfully marketing
and selling your services to
employer groups.
*Make Your Good Publicity Work
Marketing Magic!*
An audiocassette program packed
with tips and steps you can take to
cost-efficiently maximize the
marketing impact of your center's
good publicity. Learn how to
extend marketing dollars while
communicating a positive center
image.
The Enrollment Generator newsletter
is published bimonthly for $29 per
year by The Julian Group.

APPENDIX 8

FIELD OFFICES
of the
U.S. Small Business Administration

Agana, Guam	Fargo, ND	Nashville, TN
Albany, NY	Fresno, CA	Newark, NJ
Albuquerque, NM	Gulfport, MI	New Orleans, LA
Anchorage, AK	Harlingen, TX	New York, NY
Atlanta, GA	Harrisburg, PA	Oklahoma City, OK
Augusta, ME	Hartford, CT	Omaha, NE
Baltimore, MD	Hato Rey, PR	Philadelphia, PA
Birmingham, AL	Helena, MT	Phoenix, AZ
Boise, ID	Holyoke, MA	Pittsburgh, PA
Boston, MA	Honolulu, HI	Portland, OR
Buffalo, NY	Houston, TX	Providence, RI
Casper, WY	Indianapolis, IN	Rapid City, SD
Charleston, WV	Jackson, MI	Richmond, VA
Charlotte, NC	Jacksonville, FL	Rochester, NY
Chicago, IL	Kansas City, MO	St. Louis, MO
Cincinnati, OH	Knoxville, TN	Salt Lake City, UT
Clarksburg, WV	Las Cruces, NM	San Antonio, TX
Cleveland, OH	Las Vegas, NV	San Diego, CA
Columbia, SC	Little Rock, AR	San Francisco, CA
Columbus, OH	Los Angeles, CA	Seattle, WA
Concord, NH	Louisville, KY	Sioux Falls, SD
Corpus Christi, TX	Lubbock, TX	Spokane, WA
Dallas, TX	Madison, WI	Springfield, IL
Denver, CO	Marquette, MI	Syracuse, NY
Des Moines, IA	Marshall, TX	Tampa, FL
Detroit, MI	Memphis, TN	Washington, DC
Eau Claire, WI	Miami, FL	Wichita, KS
Elmira, NY	Milwaukee, WI	Wilkes-Barre, PA
El Paso, TX	Minneapolis, MN	Wilmington, DE
Fairbanks, AK	Montpelier, VT	

ATTENTION: SCHOOLS AND CORPORATIONS

Patricia Gallagher's books are available at quantity discounts for
educational, business, or sales promotional use. For information,
please write to Special Sales Department, Young Sparrow Press,
Box 265, Worcester, PA 19490

APPENDIX 9

SAMPLE STATE FORMS

The following forms are samples of those required for licensing in my home state of Pennsylvania. Forms required vary from state to state.

This is just to give you some idea of the type of information needed for state licensure.

DAY CARE SERVICES

ENROLLMENT/ATTENDANCE RECORD

MONTH _____ 19 ___

NAME	FEE	AGE	TYPE OF SVC.	1	2	3	4	5	6	7	8	9	10	11	12	13	14	15	16	17	18	19	20	21	22	23	24	25	26	27	28	29	30	31	Total Days Enrolled	Total Days Attended

NUMBER OF DAYS FACILITY WAS OPEN _____ AVERAGE DAILY ENROLLMENT _____ AVERAGE DAILY ATTENDANCE _____

TOTAL PLACED ON REGISTER _____

TOTALS _____

PW 29A - 8-81

ADMINISTRATION OF SYRUP OF IPECAC

55 PA CODE CHAPTERS 3270.75(c),3270.133(9); 3280.75(c),3280.75(9); 3290.73(c),3290.133(9)

PHYSICIAN OR POISON CONTROL MUST BE CALLED BEFORE ADMINISTERING SYRUP OF IPECAC

CHILD'S NAME	CHILD'S WEIGHT	CHILD'S AGE

AFTER THE CALL TO POISON CONTROL COMPLETE THE FOLLOWING:

INDIVIDUAL ISSUING INSTRUCTION	TIME INSTRUCTION RECEIVED	DATE INSTRUCTION RECEIVED
CONTENT OF INSTRUCTION:		

ADMINISTERED BY	TIME ADMINISTERED	DATE ADMINISTERED
AMOUNT ADMINISTERED		
ADDITIONAL COMMENTS:		

03885A

CY 865 - 1/93

IF FACILITY ADMINISTERS SYRUP OF IPECAC AN INCIDENT REPORT MUST BE COMPLETED
CHAPTERS 3270.132(C),3270.133(9); 3280.132(c),3280.133(9); 3290.132(c),3290.133(9)

VERBAL REQUEST FOR RELEASE OF CHILD

55 PA CODE CHAPTERS 3270.117(c), 3280.117(c) and 3290.116(c)

THIS FORM MUST BE COMPLETED TO DOCUMENT THE VERBAL REQUEST BY A PARENT FOR THE RELEASE OF A CHILD TO A PERSON(S) NOT INDICATED ON THE AGREEMENT
(CHAPTERS 3270.123(a)(5),3270.124(b)(7); 3280.123(a)(5),3280.124(b)(7); 3290.123(a)(5),3290.124(b)(7)).

NAME OF CHILD	DATE	TIME
NAME OF REQUESTING PARENT		
TELEPHONE NO. FROM WHICH PARENT IS CALLING		
NAME OF INDIVIDUAL TO WHOM THE CHILD IS TO BE RELEASED ▶		
NAME OF STAFF PERSON TAKING THE CALL ▶		

CALL THE ENROLLING PARENT BACK TO CONFIRM THE INFORMATION IF POSSIBLE

CONFIRMING PARENT	DATE
NAME OF STAFF PERSON CONFIRMING INFORMATION	TIME

_____   _____
NAME OF STAFF PERSON RELEASING CHILD   DATE

BE SURE TO ASK FOR IDENTIFICATION WHEN THE INDIVIDUAL ARRIVES TO PICK UP THE CHILD

MEDICATION LOG

55 PA CODE CHAPTERS 3270.133; 3280.133; 3290.133

I GIVE PERMISSION TO ADMINISTER MEDICATION TO MY CHILD AS STATED BELOW

DATE	PARENT'S SIGNATURE	CHILD'S NAME	NAME OF MEDICATION	* P/N	TIME TO BE GIVEN	AMOUNT/ DOSAGE	REFRIG REQ?	STAFF COMPLETE THIS SECTION				
								TIME GIVEN	AMOUNT/ DOSAGE	STAFF INITIALS	DATE	COMMENT/ REACTION

*P = PRESCRIPTION   N = NON-PRESCRIPTION

FIRE DRILL LOG
55 PA CODE CHAPTERS 3270.94; 3280.94; 3290.94

DATE	TIME	HYPOTHETICAL LOCATION	EVACUATION TIME	PARTICIPATING FACILITY PERSON	NUMBER OF CHILDREN

03886A

CHILD HEALTH APPRAISAL

CHILD DAY CARE CENTERS ● GROUP DAY CARE HOMES ● FAMILY DAY CARE HOMES

DATE OF EXAM

CHILD'S NAME (Last, First, M.I.)

BIRTHDATE

CHILD'S ADDRESS

TELEPHONE NUMBER

1. REVIEW OF HEALTH HISTORY

2. MEDICAL INFO. PERTINENT TO DIAG. AND TREATMENT IN CASE OF EMERGENCY

3. SPECIAL INSTRUCTIONS TO PROVIDER REGARDING ANY MEDICATION REQUIRED DURING DAY CARE HOURS

4. RECOMMENDED MODIFICATIONS OR LIMITATIONS OF CHILD'S ACTIVITIES OR DIET (e.g. allergies, etc.)

5. VISION (Acuity) ☐ Normal ☐ Abnormal

6. HEARING (Audiometry or equiv.)
Subjective Screening (Date) _____
Audiometry (Date) _____

7. GROWTH MEASUREMENT
Ht. ___ ' ___ Percentile   Wt. ___ lbs. ___ Percentile   Circ. ___ " ___ Percentile

8. DENTAL SCREENING	YES	NO
Caries		
Missing Permanent Teeth		
Oral Infection		
Protrusion		

9. MEDICAL	Normal	Abnormal		Normal	Abnormal
Ears, Nose			Abdomen		
Eyes			Genitalia, Breasts		
Mouth, Throat			Extremities/Joints		
Lungs			Spine		
Cardio-Vascular			Skin, Lymph Nodes		

10. HGB
HGB ☐ Normal ☐ Abnormal
GM OR HCT ☐ Normal ☐ Abnormal
% _____

11. BLOOD PRESSURE ▶ ___ / ___
☐ Normal ☐ Abnormal

12. DEVELOPMENTAL APPRAISAL
IS CHILD PROGRESSING NORMALLY WITH AGE OR GROUP? ☐ YES ☐ NO   DENVER DEVELOPMENTAL: ☐ Normal ☐ Abnormal

13. IMMUNIZATIONS

DTP: Diphtheria–Tetanus–Pertusis	DATE	TRIVALENT ORAL POLIO VACCINE	DATE	OTHER	DATE
1st (2 months)		1st (2 months)		Measles (15 months or older)	
2nd (4 months)		2nd (4 months)		Mumps (15 months or older)	
3rd (6 months)		3rd (18 months)		Rubella (15 months or older)	
Booster		4th (4 - 6 years)		HIB (Haemophilus b) (18 Months)	
Booster		Urinalysis		Tuberculin test	

14. RECOMMEND FURTHER MEDICAL TESTS OR EXAMINATION ON THE FOLLOWING:

☐ VISION   ☐ GROWTH   ☐ HBG   ☐ HEAD CIRCUMFERENCE   ☐ HEARING   ☐ DENTAL   ☐ BLOOD PRESSURE

☐ MEDICAL (Specify)

☐ DEVELOPMENTAL PROGRESS (Specify)

☐ IMMUNIZATION (Specify)

PRINTED NAME OF PHYSICIAN

TELEPHONE NO.

PHYSICIAN'S ADDRESS

PHYSICIAN'S SIGNATURE

DATE

SP 4-164 (3-91)

FOR CENTRAL REPOSITORY USE ONLY
(LEAVE BLANK)

PENNSYLVANIA STATE POLICE
REQUEST FOR CRIMINAL RECORD CHECK

TYPE OR PRINT LEGIBLY WITH INK

PART I   TO BE COMPLETED BY REQUESTER

DATE OF REQUEST

NAME (SUBJECT OF RECORD CHECK)
(Last)   (First)   (Middle)

MAIDEN NAME AND/OR ALIASES | SOCIAL SECURITY NO. (SOC) | DATE OF BIRTH (DOB) | SEX | RACE

- - - - - - - - - - - - - - - - - - (FOLD) - - - - - - - - - - - - - - - - - -

REASON FOR REQUEST: (CHECK APPROPRIATE BLOCK)

☐ EMPLOYMENT

☐ OTHER (SPECIFY) _____

☐ INDIVIDUAL ACCESS AND REVIEW BY SUBJECT OF RECORD CHECK
OR LEGAL REPRESENTATIVE (AFFIDAVIT OF LEGAL
REPRESENTATION ATTACHED)

REQUESTER IDENTIFICATION: (CHECK APPROPRIATE BLOCK)

☐ INDIVIDUAL/NONCRIMINAL JUSTICE AGENCY - ENCLOSE A
CERTIFIED CHECK/MONEY ORDER (NONREFUNDABLE) IN
THE AMOUNT OF $10.00 PAYABLE TO "COMMONWEALTH OF
PENNSYLVANIA".
DO NOT SEND CASH/PERSONAL CHECK.

☐ NONCRIMINAL JUSTICE AGENCY - FEE EXEMPT

INFORMATION WILL BE MAILED TO REQUESTER ONLY

LIST TELEPHONE NUMBER TO BE USED TO
CONTACT REQUESTER IF NECESSARY.

NAME OF REQUESTER

ADDRESS

(AREA CODE)

CITY   STATE   ZIP CODE

☐☐☐ - ☐☐☐ - ☐☐☐☐

NOTE:

A "NO RECORD" RESPONSE WILL TAKE TWO (2) WEEKS
TO PROCESS; A "RECORD" RESPONSE WILL TAKE LONGER.

IF THIS FORM IS NOT LEGIBLE OR PROPERLY COMPLETED, IT WILL
BE RETURNED UNPROCESSED TO REQUESTER.

- - - - - - - - - - - - - - - - - - (FOLD) - - - - - - - - - - - - - - - - - -

REQUESTER CHECKLIST:

✔ DID YOU ENTER THE FULL NAME, DOB, AND SOC?

✔ DID YOU ENCLOSE THE $10.00 FEE (CERTIFIED CHECK/MONEY
ORDER)?   DO NOT SEND CASH/PERSONAL CHECK.

✔ DID YOU ENTER YOUR COMPLETE ADDRESS INCLUDING ZIP
CODE AND TELEPHONE NUMBER IN THE BLOCKS PROVIDED?

AFTER COMPLETION MAIL BOTH COPIES WITH CARBON INTACT TO:

PENNSYLVANIA STATE POLICE CENTRAL REPOSITORY
1800 ELMERTON AVENUE
HARRISBURG, PENNSYLVANIA 17110-9758

PART II   CENTRAL REPOSITORY RESPONSE

INFORMATION DISSEMINATED:

☐ NO RECORD   ☐ CRIMINAL RECORD ATTACHED

INQUIRY/DISSEMINATED BY: | SID NO:

THE INFORMATION DISSEMINATED BY THE CENTRAL REPOSITORY IS BASED SOLELY ON THE
FOLLOWING IDENTIFIERS THAT MATCH THOSE FURNISHED BY THE REQUESTER:

☐ NAME   ☐ DATE OF BIRTH   ☐ RACE

☐ SOC   ☐ MAIDEN/ALIAS NAME   ☐ SEX

CERTIFIED BY:

(DIRECTOR, CENTRAL REPOSITORY)

Response based on comparison of data provided by the requester in Part I against information contained in the files of the Pennsylvania State
Police Central Repository only, and does not preclude the existence of other criminal records which may be contained in the repositories of other
local, state or federal criminal justice agencies.

ORDER FORM

Titles:

Start Your Own At-Home Child Care Business (Doubleday)

Includes how to advertise, promote your business, gather the right equipment and toys, licensing, insurance and zoning information, daily activities, craft recipes, no-cook baking ideas, where to obtain free supplies and much much more. An indispensable, step-by-step guidebook to help you avoid problems and improve the profit of your business. **$14.95**

So You Want To Open A Profitable Day Care Center (How To Operate A Successful Child Care Center)

Expanded, revised, more complete than ever. Explains how to begin, methods of financing, legal aspects, effective marketing techniques, tips from experienced directors, potential problems, how to avoid them. What every new and experienced director needs to be successful. The leading book in its field! **$19.95**

How To Entertain Children At Home Or In Preschool

Chock full of what to do when a child says, "There's nothing to do!" Simple crafts, learning activities, songs, games, finger plays, and free supply ideas. A wonderful resource filled with easy-to-do projects that can be made with items that don't cost a lot of money. **$14.95**

For All The Write Reasons: Forty Successful Authors, Publishers, Agents, and Writers Tell You How To Get Your Book Published

Includes how to find an interested publisher, agent, or editor; negotiate a favorable contract; have your book mentioned in newspapers and magazines; obtain favorable book reviews; appear on local and national television shows. **$21.95**

Raising Happy Kids On A Reasonable Budget

Includes inexpensive ways to feed your family, ranging from bulk buying and couponing to home gardening. How to clothe the family by haunting second-hand stores, outlets and end-of-season sales. Money-saving educational tips, including ways to cut college costs. Keeping your kids healthy and well-groomed, including thrifty advice on prescriptions and health care. Low-cost family vacations — lots of ideas to get you started. **$13.95**

SPECIAL BOOKLETS

1. Tips About Operating a Day Care Program   **$2.00**
2. 100 Ways to Keep Kids Happy   **$2.00**
3. How to Deal with Common Day Care Problems   **$2.00**

Special Booklets may be purchased individually as listed or are offered free when you buy any three of Patricia Gallagher's books. Order three books and receive all "Special Booklets" absolutely free! ($6.00 retail value).

Please expedite my order for Patricia C. Gallagher's Books:
☐ I have enclosed a check for $_____
☐ Charge the total amount due on my order to my: ☐ VISA   ☐ MasterCard

Card # _____

Expiration Date _____

Name on Card_____

Phone Number _____

Please print your complete mailing address below:

Name _____

Organization _____

Address _____

City, State, Zip _____

Phone _____

PA residents add 6% sales tax. Add $3.00 for postage and handling.
To order send to: P. Gallagher, Box 555, Worcester, PA 19490
or call (215) 364-1945.
SATISFACTION GUARANTEED OR MONEY BACK!